THE GUIDEBOOK TO
OPTIMUM
HEALTH

Why Exercise &
Nutrition Alone
Are Not Enough

CARL
MASSY

First printed in 2014
Cover design and book layout by Ferry Tan of Invisible Resources.
ISBN: 978-981-09-1408-0

For information about special discounts for bulk purchases, please contact Carl Massy at: carl@carlmassy.com.

For information about bringing Carl Massy or his team to a live event or delivering an in-depth transformational workshop, please contact Carl Massy at: carl@carlmassy.com.

Dedication

To my amazing partner, Ferry, who believes in me more than myself on the odd occasion. Thank you so much.

And to all of the amazing teachers, past and present, I have had the privilege to learn from and share experiences with — thank you for sharing your wisdom.

CONTENTS

Introduction

Nothing splendid has ever been achieved
except by those who dared believe that something
inside them was superior to circumstance.
Bruce Barton, American author, advertising executive, and politician

Today is one of my toughest days. Today I'm beginning a book that is very dear to me, and I'm excitedly nervous about starting well so you get drawn in and totally engaged.

First of all, *The Guidebook to Optimum Health* is my second book. The first was a book on happiness called (unsurprisingly), *The Guidebook to Happiness*. If you're on the second leg of this journey with me, you already know a bit about this Aussie bloke called Carl Massy. For those new to me (and perhaps the subject matter), I'll briefly summarize my background so you can get the measure of your guide on this journey to optimum health and wellbeing.

Growing up I had two hobbies: playing sports and reading books. I was fit, active and healthy. My 'junk food' consumption as a kid consisted of one glass of Coca Cola and five squares of chocolate once a week. Wow! Those crazy Friday night binges.

This healthy lifestyle continued until, at age 17, I arrived at the Australian Defence Force Academy in Canberra, Australia to begin officer training for the Australian Army. In the early days I washed my meals down with copious amounts of beer or rum—which is how I learned my first major health lesson in life: Lots of beer or rum is not great for optimum health. It also won't keep you out of hospital after you do a back somersault off a bar and nearly fracture both heels. Ouch.

I also learned about leadership—a topic I just realized is really important for the start of this book.

You see the human body is made up of about 30-40 trillion cells (not including the 100 trillion or so bacteria living in our digestive system). That's a lot of zeros and pretty hard to fathom. So is the idea that there are *billions* of biological operations happening in our bodies every second—operations the brain and the brain in action (what we call the mind) have to direct, control and manage.

All these cells and operations need good leadership and organization for the body to function optimally. And in the military I learned that the greatest leaders are those who are most capable of *creating the environment* that is most conducive for a team or a collective whole to be successful at doing what they're supposed to do. Which brings me to my point: When it comes to you and your health, YOU are the leader, not the man or woman in the white jacket at the doctor's office or local hospital.

You are the general with teams of experts at your command—teams like the circulatory system, the nervous system, the brain, the hormonal system, the lymphatic system, the immune system—teams informing and guiding those 30-40 trillion cells in your body. Having these teams at your disposal is nothing short of INCREDIBLE. And if you create the environment that is most conducive to their success, your body will have the ability to attain a state of optimum health and stay there.

Leadership is what this book is all about: Showing you what you can do, specifically, to create an environment that will allow your mind and body systems to get on with the job of rejuvenating, regenerating, and energizing your life. It's about knowing how to fully experience life with the health, vitality and energy to bring out your best. It's about fully expressing your uniqueness and making differences, big and small, on the people and world around you. It's about optimum health.

So, what do I mean by that?

Optimum health is a state of being where you rarely get sick. And if you do get sick, you're quick to recover. Just like an elite athlete's heart rate after a race, you bounce back quickly. You have high levels of vitality that give you the energy to overcome life's inevitable obstacles and move towards your most audacious goals. You have an aura about you which attracts people. Others want to be around you because it makes them feel good. (It's all a matter of something called entrainment. But we'll be talking about that later.)

Optimum health also contributes to happiness, because, let's face it, being sick sucks. Regardless of how many houses in the Caribbean you own, if you don't have your health, you're not likely to be walking around with a smile on your face and a spring in your step.

Optimum health means aging gracefully. Marshall your troops—I mean your body's biological teams—and you'll look at least 10 years younger than the number on your driver's license. You'll constantly amaze people with your age! You'll have no problems going for amazing mountain hikes through the wilderness or biking across France because your fitness levels are in good order and your body moves well and your joints and muscles are pain-free.

Headaches. What are they? Pooping problems? Not me. Colds and flu? Rarely, and definitely not for long. Major illnesses? It will seem they only happen to other people, and if something major does happen, you'll know what you need to add to your diet and your life or what to cut out in order to get on top of it.

As Wallace D. Wattles said in his book, *The Science of Getting Rich*, wealth "is about doing certain things, in certain ways." And it's the same thing with health! In this book I'll be taking you on an amazing holistic journey to understand the 6 Pillars, or six major areas of your life where by doing "certain things in certain ways" the wealth of optimum health can be yours.

It's my personal mission to help you create the environment (through knowledge and specific practices) that is most conducive to being the very best you possible. And I want to thank you now for this opportunity to share this journey with you.

I also promise to impart everything I have learned and practiced in my own quest to have the vitality and clarity of mind to fully express myself and make a positive difference for others. Which brings me back to my brief biography.

In 1999, I attended an *Unleash the Power Within* seminar with Tony Robbins which was the catalyst for picking up my first book on health and wellbeing, Deepak Chopra's *Ageless Body, Timeless Mind*. Since then, I've read over 500 books on longevity, health, wellbeing, and personal development. I've travelled the world, studied to become a personal fitness trainer, and completed Reiki masters training. I've been certified as a NLP master practitioner and hypnotherapist, and learned yoga and meditation. After leaving the army I was a security consultant to four Olympic games and one of the Asian Games.

Just like you, I've lived a diverse life. I've done stupid things and some not so stupid things. I've been a carnivore, an omnivore, a vegetarian, a vegan, and now I'm a flexitarian. I've had pneumonia, pleurisy, a knee reconstruction, appendicitis, a hernia, and a few other ailments over my life, so I know what pain and ill-health feel like and how they can take over. I've been in a very rewarding relationship for the last six years, and we have an awesome sausage dog called Apple who is sitting at me feet just now.

Bottom line, this book is an executive summary of all the great books I have read, all the courses I have attended, all the stuff I've tested personally and sweated through, and all the results I've seen with my own clients. But be assured, regardless of all the wonderful information, I also promise to keep things light and have a bit of fun along the way! You don't want to hang out with a guide who's as boring as watching paint dry. (Fortunately I have an editor who makes sure all the really bad jokes are left on the cutting room floor.)

Maybe one day we'll get to swap stories about the silly (and great) things we've done as we worked at becoming leaders of our lives and health, creating the environments most conducive to fostering greatness and wellbeing in ourselves and in all people everywhere. What a tale that will be.

Now, let's get the journey started!!

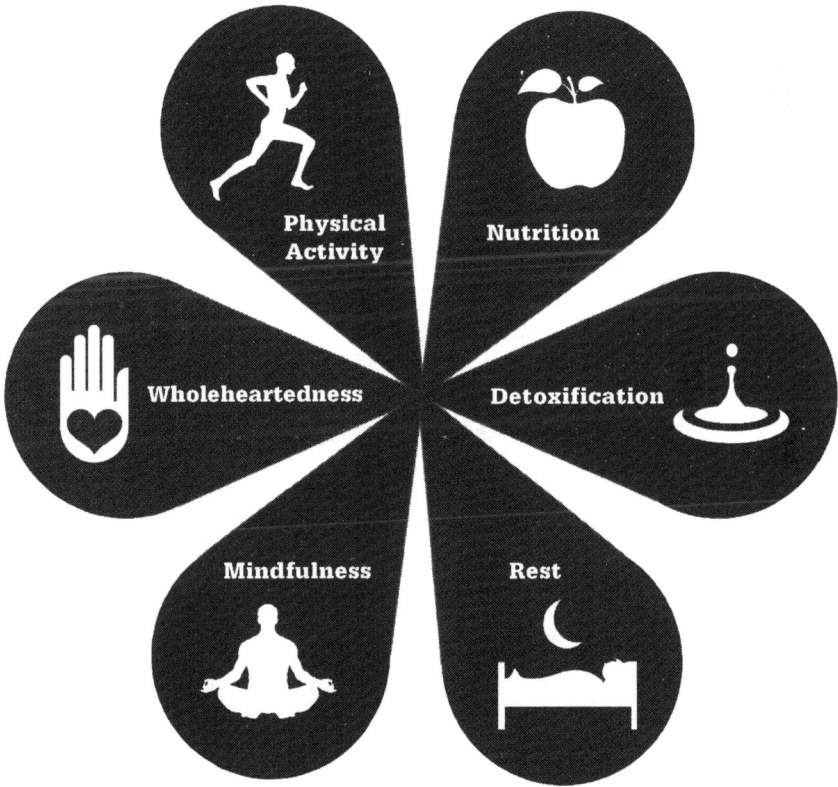

Physical Activity

Nutrition

Wholeheartedness

Detoxification

Mindfulness

Rest

CHAPTER 1:

An Optimum Health Symphony

The best time to plant a tree is twenty years ago.
The second best time is now.
Chinese Proverb

We talked about what optimum health is—being free from illness, having high levels of energy and vitality, a lightness of spirit, happiness, incredible resilience, and a long and active lifespan. But is this possible? Can you think of anyone who can tick off all of those boxes? Remember, if one person can do it, so can you!

The possibility

This level of health is definitely something to strive towards. There are people who go their whole lives without ever having spent time in the hospital or a doctor's office. One time while training, I met a girl in a Sydney gym who was in her early forties and she hadn't experienced a cold or flu since she was seven years of age. That's pretty impressive. And she's not an isolated case.

We *can* be free from illness and be a *realistic optimist* when it comes to Optimum Health. We can have high levels of energy, experience rare periods being unwell, and have an ability to bounce back quickly from any setbacks. Research shows there are also things we can do, or stop doing, which significantly affect our overall health, reducing the risk for major illnesses or diseases like coronary heart disease, diabetes, Alzheimer's, osteoporosis, and even cancer. But, as you will see, we can't get there just by doing one or two things. We have to take a HOLISTIC approach to our health.

One of the impediments to optimum health for all of us is the modern scientific orientation called *reductionism*. There is a trend in private scientific research (generally funded by big pharmaceutical companies and major corporate players in the food industry) and government bodies trying to isolate the one BIG THING: the *magic bullet* to health. They're looking for that isolated tablet, gene, vitamin, phytonutrient, or hormone which will take care of all our health issues at once and forever. Personally, I believe the magic pill does not exist (or is unlikely to exist in the foreseeable future). Why? Because quantum physics tells us interconnectedness is a happening thing. And in the health arena that means taking a holistic view, taking into account the intricacies of the body, its environment, our attitudes and other health factors. Without that orientation we're spending time, money and energy on isolated 'bullets' that do not work and often even take us backwards.

The symphony

So often scientists single out one or two things in a substance, such as an apple, that make it beneficial without realizing there's a symphony of vitamins, minerals, phytonutrients, water, fiber, and macronutrients working together in a magical way science has yet to fully understand. Which is why, when it comes to health, I like the analogy of a symphony where many individual instruments come together to create something better as a whole.

For a while I couldn't decide between The Symphony to Optimum Health or The 6 Pillars to Optimum Health. As you can see, the 6 pillars won out. The 6 pillars also represents the idea that if you remove one of them the roof they're supporting (your optimum health) is going to be compromised, and if you remove more than one the whole roof is going to come tumbling down. Plus, I worked for a couple of years in Greece with a regular view of the Acropolis. So pillars it is.

The 6 Essential Pillars for Attaining Optimum Health

Too many health programs and books on health focus only on the physical things we can do without understanding that our greatest physical efforts can be completely derailed by a mind that is not in alignment and emotions that are unprocessed or habitually negative. This book is complete and deals with all parts of ourselves in an integrated fashion: the body, the mind and our emotions. It's only when all three are congruent that we can reach our highest levels of health, vitality and active longevity.

The 6 Pillars we will be exploring in-depth together in this guidebook are:

1. Physical Activity
2. Nutrient abundance
3. Detoxification
4. Rest
5. Mindfulness
6. Wholeheartedness

Pillar 1 to Pillar 4 are all about the physical body. They include specific physical and behavioral things we can start or stop doing to achieve optimum health. Pillar 5 takes us into the realm of the mind and therefore into a place of subtle energies and consciousness. And finally, Pillar 6 takes us into the 'heart' space and those things called emotions.

Let's have a quick look at each pillar in turn before we dive into the details.

Pillar 1: Physical Activity

Many people are opposed to exercising but are cool with getting a little physical activity happening in their lives. But then I had the joy of watching a *YouTube* video featuring Ido Portal, who has dedicated his life to the practice and teaching of movement. I saw beauty and completeness in that singular word. We were born to move. It's not a maybe—it's a must. In this guide you will also discover that movement is not just about the body!

Pillar 2: Nutrient abundance

I like to get away from the terms 'diet' and even 'nutrition' because I want to focus on the key to optimum health. And the key to optimum health is increasing the quality and quantity of the health-providing nutrients you put in your body. I will be telling you exactly what those nutrients are, where you can find the little critters and also what's best to avoid—what we might call anti-nutrients.

Pillar 3: Detoxification

Unfortunately, humanity has done a pretty crappy job of taking care of the environment. I'm not here to point the finger at anyone, but the reality is we live in a world that is full of pollutants, chemicals, artificial 'food,' synthetic elements, toxins and a bunch of other stuff you don't need in your magnificent body. Scientists have no clue about the long-term effects of some foods in the supermarket on your health and wellbeing. I'm not here to scare you. I'm here to suggest there are things we can do to avoid unwanted pollutants in our bodies and also ways to remove those that have already slipped in the gates.

Pillar 4: Rest

You may be surprised to see rest here. But I can assure you, hand on heart, that you will never be at your best in health, happiness, relationships, contentment, and even success if you pay lip service to rest. There are a lot of other 'R' words associated with rest, like recovery, rejuvenation, re-creation, recreation, regeneration, and relaxation. The day before I started writing the section on rest, I did an interview with Patty Tucker, a sleep coach from the USA. I am now even more conscious of the vital role that rest plays in optimum health and optimal living.

Pillar 5: Mindfulness

I briefly explored the inner workings of the mind in *The Guidebook to Happiness*. But here I'm going to dig deeper and go into the relationship between the brain and our emotions. It took me some time to come up with a word I would use to describe this instrument in the optimum health symphony.

The mind has an incredibly powerful impact on our health. But trying to define that with one word was a challenge. In the end I chose the word 'mindfulness' because, for me, it means using the mind consciously, creatively and with purposeful intent on a consistent daily basis. As Buddha said, "We become what we think." So get ready for an amazing journey into the inner recesses of that incredibly powerful mind of yours.

Pillar 6: Wholeheartedness

For a long time there were only 5 pillars. But then I realized someone may be taking great care of their nutrition, rest, detoxification, physical activity, and even mindfulness, but still be suffering from ill-health. After listening to the great work of author and researcher Brene Brown, I realized the missing ingredient was 'wholeheartedness.'

Here is a classic example of what happens when we approach health without considering the whole—the whole, in this case, being life itself. You can tick off all the other boxes (or pillars), but if you are in a toxic relationship, doing a job you hate, feeling isolated or disconnected, the adverse effect on your health is immense. You cannot experience optimum health if you are not happy and fulfilled in your life. You cannot be wholehearted. You can only be half-hearted. And who can experience health with half a heart?

This is a Guidebook

The last point I want to make is, this is not the *10 Commandments to Optimum Health*. It's *The Guidebook to Optimum Health*. It's not about rules. It's about getting conscious and making different choices.

A guidebook is extremely valuable when you're traveling to a foreign country. But it is not the journey. Following the suggestions the guidebook provides is what determines if you have a great experience or not. You know what you like. You know what works best for you. Well, I'm just like Fodor's. I'm providing a guide to the things that research and my own experiences have taught me will provide the highest probability of optimum health. But the journey is up to you.

Second, I am not a doctor. I just care greatly for my health. I don't want okay health. I want GREAT health and high levels of energy; I want to feel extremely alive and vital; I want my body to function optimally; I want to be happy on the journey, which, as you know, is difficult if your health is crap.

Rather than focusing on illness, which is mostly what modern medicine does, over the last 15 years I've focused on the Big Question of 'what constitutes great health?' What are healthy, happy people doing? What are they eating? What does their lifestyle look like? What has been consistently verified as being good for health and happiness? What works in different countries and cultures? It's these questions, and others like them, that give us a great picture of how to stay on the healthy side of life.

And finally, life still remains a mystery for us all. Quantum physics tells us that observation and intention, thoughts and emotions and attitudes affect life at the quantum level - meaning we have a lot more influence on our lives and bodies than we imagined. Epigenetics also states that emotions and attitudes and the external environment color the expression of the genes in our DNA. And we pass these attitudes and expressions directly to our children genetically. Obviously, where we put our attention, the awareness we maintain, and the quality of the choices we make are vastly important.

I encourage you to be open throughout this journey—open with me (your guide), and open to your powerful innate intelligence and this thing called 'life' which weaves its magic around us as we get into the flow of doing what is healthy for us, healthy for others, and healthy for the greater good.

Here's to learning and new experiences and trusting life on this path to optimum health. Time to enjoy the ride!

CHAPTER 2:

Supporting Tools

If you've read *The Guidebook to Happiness* you know I like to track things. I like to create and use tools. I like to be strategic in how I present information so you get the most benefit as I'm inspiring you into action. Not big actions that change the world in a day. I want to inspire you to take small actions that change you each and every day so you become a greater expression of you.

Did you know that if you meditate (or do relaxation exercises) for five minutes every day for 365 days that you will have meditated for 1825 minutes? That's not only impressive, it will evolve your mind in all the right ways.

Old Lao Tzu told us, "The journey of 1000 miles starts with one step." I am here to help you take that first step towards optimum health. Plus give you a gentle shove if that's what is needed. Or, if you're already walking the path to optimum health, I'm going to help you put even more spring in your step, adding years of quality time to your life.

Now, back to supporting tools. I strongly recommend that you honor yourself and the value of this journey by recording where you are now. As a consultant to the Olympic Games Committee, I realized it was always important for a client to understand exactly where their start point was for a number of reasons:

1. You want to know what you're working with.
2. You want to know where your strengths are, so you can capitalize on them.
3. You want to know where your weaknesses are so you can build these up.

4. You can't celebrate your success at how far you've come if you don't mark where you started.

So, here is the first tracking tool to help you become an optimum health strategist working on the most important and priceless project of your life — Project You!

Please complete the table below to track exactly where you think you are in relation to the 6 Optimum Health Pillars.

	1	10	Rating
Physical Activity	Not happening.	6 days a week. Mixed activities. Good knowledge.	
Rest	Always tired. Restless sleep. Never stop.	Sleep deeply and well. Take breaks often. Relaxed.	
Nutrition	Terrible diet and you know it.	Only healing foods pass by your lips.	
Detoxification	Don't even know what it means.	Practice it daily, weekly and yearly.	
Mindfulness	A zombie and completely reative.	A Zen master.	
Wholeheartedness	Life is a train wreck.	In line to be the next Dalai Lama.	

Do your best to make an objective assessment of where you believe you fall in each of these categories. Then, I suggest you pay EXTRA attention to the Pillars that are specific to your greatest weaknesses. Do not be discouraged. The whole point is to improve! Remember, you can get better at anything you put your mind to. Your capacity to change is not based on intelligence and it is NOT FIXED. It all depends on the amount of effort you put in.

Here's a quick personal example. I like to think that I'm rather intelligent (and slightly amusing). I've also been living in Indonesia for over six years. However, my grasp of the Indonesian language is pitiful at best. This is not because I'm stupid. I've just put very little effort into learning the language. All of my business is done in English, and working on the business has been the major focus of my energy and attention.

So, if you score 'low' in any of the 6 pillars, don't take it personally. It's just a yellow flag indicating 'more focus and effort required here.' And, like I said, I'm here to help by providing you with the knowledge, the tools, the inspiration and the odd shove if you need it.

Your own Personal Journal

Now, the other tool I've put a bunch of effort into producing for you is a Personal Journal. PLEASE … USE IT!

Do yourself a favor and at your earliest convenience, check out the following website:
www.theguidebooktooptimumhealth.com

DO IT! You can thank me later.

CHAPTER 3:

Some basic principles for the journey

Pareto's Principle

Pareto's Principle, or the 80/20 rule, states that in most situations 20 percent of actions taken account for 80 percent of the results. This applies to most areas of life. For instance, we wear 20 percent of our clothes 80 percent of the time, and we use 20 percent of the programs on our computers 80 percent of the time. In business 20 percent of our clients provide 80 percent of the revenue.

Applying the 80/20 Principle to Optimum Health means there are certain things we can do that not only optimize our health, but that actually constitute 80 percent of our overall health. In other words, there are things we can do that have a much higher return on investment. And this is the nature of the information I'm sharing with you. I'm not telling you to do everything. I'm teaching you how to do the things that provide the greatest possible return for the least amount of time, energy, effort, and resources.

99 Percent Is a Bitch

Have I got your attention? Good. Now here's the first Great Tip.

This principle comes from some great work by Jack Canfield, one of the co-authors of *The Chicken Soup for the Soul* series. Jack (I prefer first names) made the statement, "99 percent is a bitch and 100 percent is a breeze."

What he's suggesting is that it's actually easier to commit to removing something 100 percent from your life than it is to remove it 99 percent of the time. This is true for two reasons:

1. When we decide to remove something 99 percent of the time, it's very hard to discern the situations when the one percent applies. And very soon the one percent turns into two percent, and then five percent and suddenly we went from 'hardly ever doing something' to actually doing it quite often. Eventually, this takes us backward.

2. If we open ourselves up the possibility of doing something or having something one percent of the time, we actually need to make a decision every time to establish if this is the one percent of the time where we're going to break our 'general rule.' From a neuroscience perspective, the decision-making process—where we use the neocortex part of our brain—is one of the biggest bioenergy consumers. So we want to conserve that mental faculty until we really need it.

Let me use Brian Johnson, the creator of *Philosophers Notes* and founder of the Entheos Academy, as a perfect example. Brian said that, as part of his nutritional goals, he wanted to stop eating at McDonald's. But when he set the goal it was not a 100 percent commitment, it was a 99 percent commitment. This is the 'almost never' commitment. But what he found was, each time he drove past a McDonald's he would be asking himself if this was the 'one-off' time he would make an exception. It became a mental struggle and test of will every time he made a pass. After going to the dark side on too many occasions, he decided he would never (100 percent of the time) eat at McDonald's. After that, there was no decision to be made. No Inner Fight Club going on. It became a no-brainer. He was now the person who did not eat at McDonald's.

There are a few things in this book I highly recommend you make a 100 percent commitment to do or not do. And when we get to them I will tell you what they are.

What Do You Value Most?

In *The Guidebook to Happiness* I included a chapter on Values (Chapter 11) and a tool I use called *Values-Based Decision Making*. I suggested that when it comes to decision-making, you really want to make decisions that are in alignment with your highest values. So my question to you is:

When it comes to your highest values, where do health and vitality sit?

If *health and vitality* are not in your Top 3 (which may be unlikely if you're reading this book), it's going to make it much harder to commit to a program of introducing new habits and removing unhealthy ones. If values like financial wealth, fame, beauty, success, relationships, recognition, and freedom, come in above it, you might have to do a little 'Value Raising' exercise with me here.

I suggest doing it straight away, rather than coming back later.

The best way to raise the value you put on your health and vitality is by coming up with lots of emotionally powerful reasons why it is SO important to you, linking each reason to your higher values.

For example, if one of my top values is financial wealth, the reason why I should work hard on my health is that it's going to help me express that value. So I'd write: '*The more health and energy I have, the more effectively I will be able to inspire my team, put in the effort I need to succeed, and power through any obstacles I have along the way.*'

So, what are the reasons increasing your health and vitality is **an absolute MUST** for you?

Have a think about it and if you really want a gold star, you can stop now or when you finish reading and answer that question fully.

Great! You're almost ready to get into *The Guidebook to Optimum Health* and take your health and your life to a whole new level.

CHAPTER 4:

Great information but how do I make myself do it?

When I started writing I was undecided where I would put this gem on *willpower*. I was going to include it in the Mindfulness Pillar because it relates mostly to the brain. In the end I realized it was something you need to know about much sooner. It's no good knowing the information and insights I share if you don't have the willpower to make it happen. For instance, you may know, without a shadow of a doubt, that movement is important for your health. But is that enough to make you get moving five days a week?

So, first a quick lesson on *willpower*.

Willpower basics
Brain Stuff

The base camp for your willpower is in the most evolved part of your brain— the pre-frontal cortex. This is the part of the brain that gives us the ability to 'Respond' consciously versus 'React' to stimuli, which is what most of the other species on the planet are limited to. We have the ability to self-reflect and choose our responses – to put the cookie back in the jar (or not open it in the first place). It allows us to see the longer-term picture (and consequences) and decide to delay instant gratification for a longer-term goal—a goal that is really nothing more than a picture or ideal we have formed in our head. Pretty amazing stuff really.

Willpower Versus IQ

In the book Succeed by Dr. Heidi Grant Halvorson, a psychologist and leading researcher on goal-setting, she cites an experiment where researchers found that a child's willpower was a bigger predictor of future success than IQ. Because our lives are greatly determined by the quality of the choices we make, the person who is able to exercise willpower and not be unhinged by the lure of short term gain is likely to make better overall choices that stack up to a much higher long-term gain in life.

Working out

The neocortex requires a lot of energy to perform optimally, and using willpower is a big drain on the brain and our energy as we confront daily choices. Do I do X or Y? Do I go this way or that way? Do I solve this challenge like this or that? Do I use this analogy or that analogy? Do I go to sleep now or later? Do I eat this food now, or another food later? This is a lot of work for the brain!

Interestingly, it turns out that our brains work similarly to other muscles in our bodies. The more you exercise your willpower the stronger it gets. And, just like a muscle, it requires adequate fuel in the form of glucose to operate (the brain uses about 20 percent of the fuel that comes into our bodies). And here's the most important point: just like a muscle, if we overuse it, it becomes temporarily weakened.

What does this teach us?

1. It's important to keep working on building up your willpower muscles. Start with the little things and then move onto the bigger stuff. Brian Johnson, CEO of Entheos, a company that helps people optimize their lives, said when he starts coaching clients one of the first tasks he sets them is to floss their teeth daily. He figures if they can't commit to doing the smaller stuff, they'd be hard pressed to do the bigger stuff. In effect, he was building up their willpower muscles.

2. We need adequate fuel if we expect our willpower to work effectively, and this means adequate glucose in our blood. Now, before you go off

and slam down the nearest high-glucose drink or soda, as you will soon learn, there are good, bad, and better choices when it comes to fuel. My recommendation is something natural with fiber and packed with nutrients – like a piece of fruit, a carrot, or some nuts. This allows a slow and constant release of glucose into your bloodstream and a more regulated supply of fuel for the mind. The other fuel you definitely need to fire up the willpower is water. Over 75 percent of the brain is made of water, and if this runs low your ability to think and use willpower goes with it.

3. If we use our willpower all day and aren't refueling, resting, and refocusing, we're likely to get to a stage where our willpower muscles are completely shot. Keep this up for days, weeks, and months, and you can imagine the end result. Someone at this point is 'burnt out' and hardly able to choose what clothes to wear.

Let me share a couple of scenarios with you.

Consider Oprah Winfrey. She's intelligent, intuitive, resilient and also has access to the best resources, teachers and information available. She also has incredible willpower. (You do not create a multi-billion dollar business empire with no willpower!) However, when it comes to her weight, she's fluctuated greatly over the years. So, what might the missing key be? Perhaps she uses so much energy and willpower on a daily basis running her many and varied businesses that when it comes time to take care of herself, her willpower muscles are fatigued.

Here's another common scenario. You've organized the kids and pickups, been in and out of meetings, replied to challenging emails, worked on a new project, dealt with new people and chewed on how to resolve an issue with your partner—and that was just before lunch! By the end of the day you're frazzled.

On the way home you drop into the supermarket for supplies. What do you think your chances are of not buying that quick fix, energy-boosting, sugar-loaded, power drink or chocolate bar your mind and body are screaming for? Your willpower is running on empty and you have two chances of bypassing the quick hit—none and bugger all!

The solution? Take a ten-minute break before you get to the supermarket—five minutes doing some breathing exercises and five minutes to eat an apple and some raw almonds.

It flows

The final (cool) point I'd like to make about willpower is based on research by social psychologists which suggests as we improve our willpower in one area of our life, it actually spills over into other areas. As you strengthen your brain's willpower potential, you gain heightened willpower in ALL areas of your life. As Kelly McGonigal, a Stanford University Professor, puts it in her book *The Willpower Instinct*: "Studies have found that committing to any small, consistent act of self-control—improving your posture, squeezing a handgrip every day to exhaustion, cutting back on sweets, and keeping track of your spending—can increase overall willpower. And while these small self-control exercises may seem inconsequential, they appear to improve the willpower challenges we care about most, including focusing at work, taking good care of our health, resisting temptation, and feeling more in control of our emotions."

In summary

Here are the key points:

1. You (yes you!) can build up your willpower, little by little.
2. To have more willpower your brain needs to be rested, hydrated and adequately fuelled (with complex carbohydrates – the opposite of junk food).
3. If you are not well-rested, hydrated and fueled, avoid putting yourself in a position where you need to exercise willpower (to either do or don't do

something). This is a HUGE key to success.

4. Practice the little stuff that Kelly suggests such as improving your posture, cutting back on sweets, etcetera.

5. Willpower is not a fixed character trait. It can be learned, practiced and expanded. Like I said, you CAN build up your willpower.

CHAPTER 5:

Getting perspective on the gene thing

I recently was asked the question, "With modern medicine today there are many tests you can have to see if you are more likely to develop some awful disease such as Huntington's and Alzheimer's. Would you want to know?" I posted the response on my blog. But I also want to share it here because a lot of people seem to think they're a slave to 'bad genes.' And if you think that, not only might you quit before you get started on the road to optimal health, you might be creating the environment in your body that takes you just where you don't want to go.

The right question

One of the things I teach on the 30-Day Happiness Challenge is to ask better questions. And also to make sure the question we are asking does not presuppose a 'fact' that is not really a fact (a fact is 100% true, 100% percent of time). Otherwise the answer we get will not be relevant. It's easy to accept the idea that, "I'm genetically predisposed to___ (fill in the blank) as 'fact' because it sounds scientific. But, as you will see, there are a lot of scientific 'facts' that don't take more holistic considerations into account.

It's important to see the larger picture, especially when it comes to health concerns. So let's take a look at this gene thing.

Genetics and epigenetics

A simple explanation of genetics is: DNA is the detailed blueprint for building cells, genes are the coded parts of the DNA that create different proteins that build the body's cells, regulating all the tissues and organs, and RNA is what copies and transmits the genes' codes to the proteins.

The important thing to know is that when proteins are created off the RNA script, the end result is not a 100 percent match to the original DNA because of *epigenetic* modifications which turn genes on or off, affecting how cells "read" genes and thus function. Okay, that's enough of the biology stuff before I confuse myself too!

But what could possibly affect our genes?

Epigenetic means "above genetics." And epigenetic changes are caused by the environment in and around each cell. In layman's terms, that means everything in our cells' environment, from external toxins introduced into the body through pollution and the foods we eat, to internally produced toxins created from stressful thoughts. All of these things *change our cells*.

Negative thoughts trigger emotions that literally shape our bodies by causing our brains to produce different molecules called neurotransmitters, neuropeptides and hormones that get released into the bloodstream. These "molecules of emotion," as they're called by Dr. Candace Pert who wrote the amazing book *Molecules of Emotion*, bind to receptor sites in cells, affecting them in different ways. Constantly repeated negative emotions, like anger or depression, literally switch off your cells' ability to receive anything but the peptides released by anger or depression. The result? You can't feel joy or happier emotions anymore.

At the same time this toxic molecular soup affects the RNA, which then affects the genes. The result? Mutated genes and illnesses like cancer.

The good news is there are tons of things we can do, or stop doing, to stimulate production of positive molecules of emotion, switch your cells' receptor sites back on and help maintain the healthy expression of our genes. American political author Norman Cousins, professor of Medical Humanities at the University of California, literally laughed his way back to health after being diagnosed with heart disease by watching Charlie Chaplin and Marx Brothers movies for hours everyday!

The placebo effect

The placebo effect is considered to be a major player in the success of most drugs. Anywhere from 30 to 100 percent of the healing results from medications can be attributed to the patient's *belief* in the ability of the drug to heal their condition. Dr. Bruce Lipton cites a medical case in his book *The Biology of Belief*, where the placebo effect worked in minor knee surgery. For one test group the medical staff pretended to do surgery by making incisions, splashing water around, talking as they would during a normal knee surgery and then sewing patients up. The fake surgery test group and the test groups who had real knee surgery received the same rehabilitation program. To everyone's surprise the fake surgery was as effective as the real surgery.

Here's the thing on modern medicine. It's EXCELLENT at treating symptoms or broken stuff, but not so great at the preventative or creating optimum health stuff. (For more on this specifically you might want to read *Mind Over Medicine* by Dr. Lissa Rankin.)

Thousands of people have cured themselves of cancer (there is a book called *Spontaneous Remission* which lists 3,500 cases), and from my research I know Alzheimer's is positively influenced by a quality diet, physical activity, regular use of mental faculties (doing mental push-ups so to speak) and other things.

So, here's the kicker. Knowing what we now know about epigenetics and the placebo effect, as you can see, the story often told by the establishment like, "there is no cure for cancer," or "Alzheimer's runs in your genes" can be hugely damaging. Believing these stories can potentially create the cellular environment that might make the stories come true.

One of the best books you are likely to read on the placebo effect is by Dr Joe Dispenza, called *You Are The Placebo*. Put it on your reading list, as you are going to love it. He has gone deeper, broader and very scientifically into not only understanding the placebo effect, but also how to tap into this intelligent power consciously and deliberately.

Worry

Which brings me around to worry.

As we have seen, medical doctors do their best. But they're not gods. There's a lot they know and do well, and a lot they don't know and don't do well. Worrying about a diagnosis or prognosis, which, in many cases is just a 'best guess,' does nothing to improve your health.

Worrying leads to the activation of the stress response, which leads to a fight or flight reaction, the release of unhealthy levels of cortisol and adrenaline into the bloodstream, and a deactivation of the immune system. Among other things, worry can lead to a breakdown, overuse, or confusion of the body's natural defenses—defenses that ensure the body runs optimally.

My hypothesis on hereditary diseases

Here's my personal theory on the hereditary thing:
- The disease might be more about beliefs (thought patterns) and the placebo effect, as opposed to a mutated gene (which is rare).
- Our thinking, emotional patterns and habitual behaviors, much of which we've learned from our family, affect our health and how our genes are expressed (epigenetics).

- We have the potential to learn new ways of thinking, feeling and behaving, which will change the expression of our genes.
- What we DO NOW matters more than grandpa's genes or the style of jeans that he wore. (ha!)
- There are 1000s of reported cases of people going into spontaneous remission—so I believe body intelligence is more impressive than the intelligence of our currently known science.

In essence: worry less and DO more.

In summary

This was a great question and a subject I think has a LOT of misinformation surrounding it—which is the problem with a reductionist perspective. Specialization is great and allows the uncovering of some amazing advancements in science. But, unless discoveries are placed against the backdrop of the whole, the bigger picture is lost. My intention for the rest of the book is to look at ALL the parts that constitute the holistic picture of body, mind, emotions and spirit.

CHAPTER 6:

S t r e s s s s s s s s

I realized I could not write a book about optimum health without addressing the subject of stress. Stress is managed and minimized by the application of all 6 Pillars, and I will be talking about it more as it relates to each. But for now, let's look at the bigger picture.

I was going to talk about stress as a big scary thing, but actually, for many of us, it is not big, nor is it scary, nor is it something we are easily and consciously aware of. It is often small, persistent, cumulative, undetectable, evasive, pervasive, and as damn sneaky as that soundless mosquito in the middle of the night. On the other hand, stress is very useful in the right doses, in the right situation, and at the right time.

Obviously we're dealing with something that is paradoxical in nature from both a positive and a negative point of view.

Are you ready for an Evolution Lesson?

I love reading about how we evolved as a species—how, once upon a time, we lived in caves, had weapons that a modern 8-year-old could make, and had their lives threatened on a regular basis by scary animals like sabre toothed tigers— which animal I will use for today's lesson.

Back in the day when a sabre toothed tiger attacked primitive man or woman, the situation would unconsciously activate the sympathetic nervous system, also known as the fight or flight response. Their bodies would release adrenalin, cortisol and norepinephrine into their bloodstream, and their blood would be directed to their major running and fighting muscles, withdrawing from the digestive organs and any other areas related to long-term repair work. The immune system would also be turned off.

The body (and mind) was dealing with something immediate and terrifying and only the relevant fight or flight body functions needed to be activated.

Our primitive person would then run or rumble with the predator and, if they survived, their body would have expended much of the stress hormones pumping through their bloodstream. Getting back to the cave, they would return to a more rested state where their body would clear any remaining stress hormones from the blood, return to digesting food (as opposed to being digested as food) and doing the repair and recovery work it was designed for.

Fast-forward thousands of years to 2014 and we see a similar, but different, thing occurring. The boss comes into your workspace and hands you additional work you're unfamiliar with that has an unrealistic deadline. What happens? Millions of years of evolution for the survival and procreation of the human race kick in.

Without any conscious thought, your mind and body move into the old 'fight or flight' program. You have a surge of stress hormones. Blood flow is redirected to different parts of your body. Your higher creative mental faculties and your brain get less blood and oxygen because you're all set to run or rumble.

Unfortunately, unlike the saber tooth tiger scenario, the solution in this case calls for you to work longer hours, get less rest, make more phone calls, send more emails, do more research, and a whole host of other very unphysical activities. This means the extra stress hormones in your bloodstream don't get utilized as nature intended. Instead they remain circulating in your system. If this continues over time with no physical release and no chance to process the hormones; if stress continues without enough time spent in a relaxed state (in your cave) to clear your blood, this will lead to chronic illness.

It doesn't take much to trigger the fight or flight response in our bodies. The above situation could just as easily been triggered by:

- A call from the school to say your child is in trouble
- An unexpected bill
- A visit from a monster-in-law (if you drew the wrong straw)
- A car breaking down
- A traffic jam on your way to an important meeting or to pick up the kids
- A cooking disaster before the dinner guests arrive
- A business meeting that goes pear-shaped

What we are left with?

This leaves us with a big challenge. Our bodies have not yet evolved to the point where a PSYCHOLOGICAL threat no longer triggers a PHYSICAL response. And we are faced with more and more psychological triggers and pressures every day.

Marketers convince us we need more and more useless things to be satisfied, which means we need to make more and more cold hard cash (or go into more and more debt) to have them. Cell phones, iPads and iPods compete for our mental attention hundreds of times a day (and night). Going from house to car to office to car and then back to our homes, we're becoming disconnected from nature. We're encouraged to achieve and perform at a higher level in not just one area, but all areas of our lives. Actually, just writing about this now was causing me to feel a little stressed until I decided to laugh at the ludicrousness of it all. (I suggest a good chuckle right now for you too!)

My point is, if stress persists on a chronic and persistent basis it will undoubtedly lead to major illness and even death. (Not the box any of us want to be ticking any time soon.) Which makes it even more important to do the things that can mitigate these high levels of stress, like some of these for example:

- Performing consistent physical activity
- Getting adequate rest
- Making superior nutritional choices
- Detoxifying your body and environment
- Practicing enhanced mindfulness techniques
- Taking care of the 'life issues' that slowly erode our health

The flip side of the coin

As an impartial judge, I also have to stand up for stress. As with everything in life, there is no absolute good or bad, right or wrong. There are two sides to every coin, and stress can actually be our friend.

We absolutely need some stress in our lives to achieve what I call 'getting shit done.' Please pardon my French messieurs and madams, but stress at the right time in the right dose for a finite period of time is definitely required to achieve things in our lives. Sometimes we need that adrenalin hit to get what we want in life. The fine line is to make sure your stress levels aren't off the Richter Scale and do not persist for extended periods of time.

Here's an example from my former Army days…

I was on the Army boxing team. After months of training when I stepped into the ring for the first time — which was a truly petrifying event — I could definitely say my body was coursing with adrenalin. This lead to tension and then fatigue in a relatively short period of time. By the second round of our 3-round match my gloves felt like they were made out of lead and my arms felt like they were moving in slow motion. The next time I fought, several years later, I was more relaxed, less full of adrenalin (stress) and light as a feather.

I also won in about one-minute and quickly retired from my amateur boxing career whilst on top.

Stress is necessary—but not too much for too long.

The autonomic nervous system

Now, let's take your education into optimum health to an even deeper level. Don't worry. There are only a couple simple diagrams to follow.

The autonomic nervous system governs automatic body functions like heart rate, digestion, respiration rate, sexual arousal, etcetera. Generally it works unconsciously. Note two points here: 1) I say *generally* because there are cases where Indian yogis and other mind-body experts can override the system and do crazy stuff like reducing their heart rate to near zero while remaining conscious; and 2) it is our thoughts, feelings and behaviour that determine how this system functions.

What follows is a diagram that shows the autonomic nervous system and its two primary sub-systems:

1. the sympathetic nervous system (fight or flight), and
2. the parasympathetic nervous system (recovery and rejuvenation)

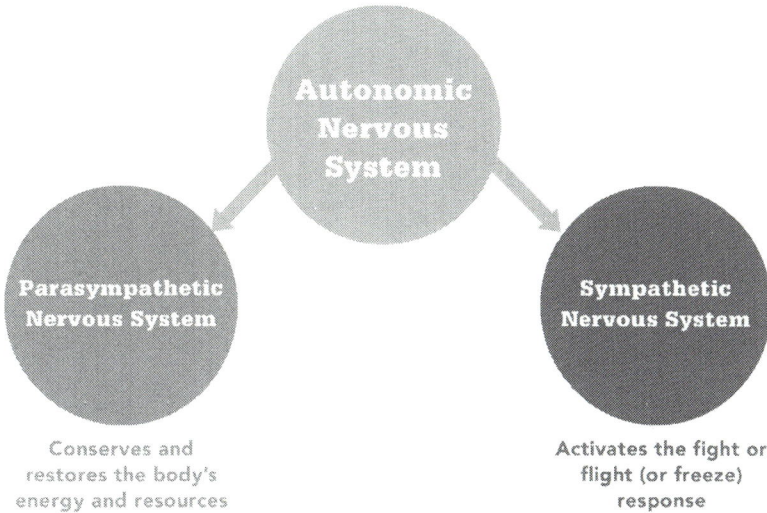

Autonomic Nervous System

Parasympathetic Nervous System

Sympathetic Nervous System

Conserves and
restores the body's
energy and resources

Activates the fight or
flight (or freeze)
response

Diagram of Autonomic Nervous System

The Sympathetic Nervous System causes physiological responses like redirecting blood flow and producing adrenaline. It also damps down the parasympathetic responses. Like our immune system, it's all about getting stuff done now.

The parasympathetic nervous system, on the other hand, is responsible for the repair and recovery work that enables us to remain in the optimum health zone. Unfortunately, cellular repair does not happen when we're in a stressed state of mind. So the longer the stressed state persists, the less time the body has to rejuvenate and regenerate.

Because our brain and nervous system have not yet evolved to the point where they no longer overreact to psychological stressors, we have to learn how to consciously direct our minds and bodies to a healing zone when this kind of stress occurs.

For optimum health, vitality, happiness and longevity, we need to spend more of our time activating the parasympathetic nervous system by doing specific things, like doing mindfulness exercises and taking planned rest breaks. Next is a diagram representing where, I believe, optimum health resides within the autonomic nervous system continuum.

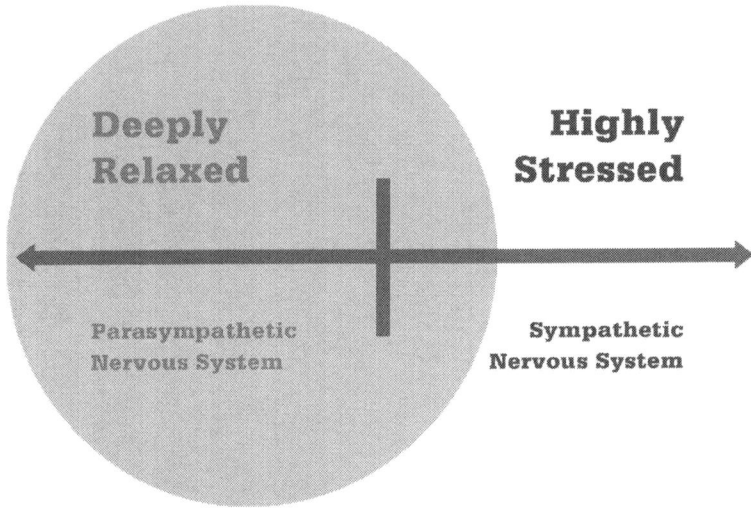

Deeply Relaxed

Highly Stressed

Parasympathetic Nervous System

Sympathetic Nervous System

Diagram of Optimum Health Zone on the Automic Nervous System Continuum

Getting ready for the road ahead

One of the key things I'm helping you to master through *The Guidebook to Optimum Health* is the detrimental effect of the tremendous amounts of stress we're subject to in this modern world. We will revisit this topic again and again from different directions as we move through the 6 Pillars.

Speaking of which, we're now ready to start the main part of this workbook. So buckle your seatbelts and get ready to learn at a super-practical level the DO's and DON'Ts when it comes to your health, your energy levels, your vitality and your ability to live a long, full, exuberant and engaged life.

Next stop—Pillar number one.

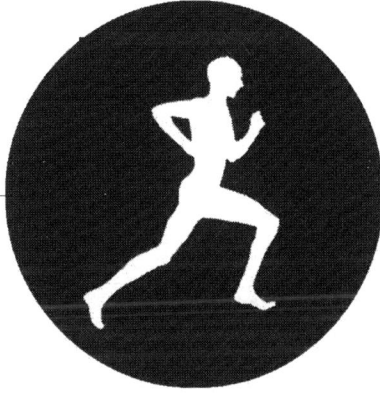

PILLAR 1
PHYSICAL ACTIVITY

Lack of activity destroys the good condition of every human being, while movement and methodical physical exercise save it and preserve it.
Plato, Greek Philosopher and mathematician

CHAPTER 7:

Why Physical Activity is so damn important!

Perhaps you're thinking, "Yeah, right. News flash. Exercise is good for me. Tell me something I don't know." And you're right. This is not cutting-edge news. But I don't want you to just know this. I want to draw on my amazing storytelling abilities and give you the down and dirty details of how vital movement is so that if I tried to drag you away from your boxfit aerobics class you'd fill the room with screams and upper-cuts.

Forget 'exercise.' Movement is life! Anything where you move the body, elevate your heart rate, huff and puff, push or pull against some sort of resistance, twist and turn, jump, slide, reach, stride, and generally break out in a sweat is the 'it' I want you chiseling out precious time in your week for. And if you're after a three-minute five days a week for six-weeks workout that will create bulging muscles you're reading the wrong book. If you want to look and feel fabulous at any age, live longer, improve your cognitive functioning and minimize wear and tear on your body while radiating real beauty from the inside out … you've come to the right place.

A wee history lesson

As little as 50 years ago, life took some 'elbow grease.' To get things done, people had to exert physical effort. To get something from the corner store they walked or cycled. To do the washing they stirred, splashed, wrung-out and hung-out their laundry. They walked up stairs. They opened doors with their bare hands. They scrubbed things. They whisked, stirred and ground ingredients to make a cake. They played games that required the movement of their whole body (as opposed to a couple of fingers). They walked to the other side of the office to have a conversation.

I'm sure you get the idea—people actually moved their bodies as part of daily life—what we now call 'incidental exercise.' But even this is a thing of the past for most people today. Which is all the more reason to pay attention to what I'm about to share with you.

The biggest why's

Optimum health IS NOT about meeting your true love at the gym while working out. Yes, it'd be a great byproduct. But the main reason you're there is because you're a human being that evolved in such a way that without physical action you function rather poorly—essentially the opposite of optimum health.

One of the biggest reasons to move the body regularly is to maintain the healthy functioning of the lymphatic system. The lymphatic system is a key part of the circulatory system and a major player in the immune system. It distributes nutrients throughout the body, keeps tissues from swelling and removes toxins. Unlike blood, which is transported through the body by that pump called the heart, the transportation of lymph fluid (and white blood cells) relies heavily on the contraction of skeletal muscles during movement. So you've got to move to maintain this vital system for optimum health.

Another big reason to move our bodies regularly is because it increases cognitive functioning of the brain. Yep, breaking a sweat makes you smarter.

In the book *Spark: How exercise will improve the performance of your brain*, authors Eric Hagerman and Dr John J. Ratey make the following observation: "It (physical activity) fosters neuroplasticity. The best way to guard against neurodegenerative diseases is to build a strong brain. Aerobic exercise accomplishes this by strengthening connections between your brain cells, creating more synapses to expand the web of connections, and spurring newly born stem cells to divide and become functional neurons in the hippocampus."

Neuroplasticity is the new buzzword in the field of neuroscience. Essentially it means the brain can change, grow new connections, rewire old connections and continue to evolve at any age. We are not born with an unchangeable brain, and, with the right lifestyle habits, we can change our brains for the better.

Want proof? Hagerman and Ratey compared the results of two groups of students taking a test. One group exercised before the exam and the other did not. The group that did physical activity before the exam got significantly higher test results than the group that did not exercise!

Want more reasons movement is essential? Here's a list Hagerman and Ratey provide of other benefits:
1. Strengthening of the cardiovascular system
2. Improvement of insulin regulation
3. Reduction of obesity and its metabolic side affects
4. Elevation of your stress threshold (and resilience)
5. Boosting the immune system
6. Increasing bone density
7. Increasing motivation

Want more reasons to get off that sofa? Research shows that following an exercise regime over a period of weeks is often as effective as drugs in treating depression over the same period of time. Tal Ben-Sharar, a leader in the field of positive psychology and former professor at Harvard University, says that, "*not exercising is like taking a depressant.*" That got your attention? It definitely got mine.

And remember, on top of all this, physical activity burns off the stress hormones we inevitably build up in our bodies. Can you say this is a slam-dunk MUST for us all?

CHAPTER 8:

What? When? How Much?

There are bazillions of different opinions about what is 'optimum exercise,' and people will cite all manner of scientific literature to support their case. Why listen to me?

Sure, I've been actively involved in physical training for 30+ years. I've done thousands of training sessions. I've worked as a personal fitness trainer. I've read a ton of literature and tried numerous different systems to find what works best. But, unlike most trainers, I'm not just after fitness. As you know, I come from the perspective of optimum health.

For over a decade I've focused on how to keep people (and myself) free of injury and pain, living longer with more vitality, ready to partake in unplanned physical activities at any moment. Which, when you stop to think about it, is really something.

How many people could, at the drop of a hat, accept an invitation to go water skiing or cross-country skiing, take a trek in the Himalayas or canoe down a river in Guatemala with the minimum preparation needed to ensure their safety from injury? That's the place of optimum health I want you to get to.

Given differing lifestyles, body shapes, resources, commitments, existing injuries or disabilities, I do not profess to have all the answers for everybody.

I can only tell you what I've learned and what I recommend for maintaining a great base level of fitness. From there it's your responsibility to find the activities that best fit your lifestyle and the specific results you're after.

Personal (and painful) experiences have taught me that before getting involved in a sport it's best to take lessons first. I tore my anterior cruciate ligament (ACL) with a spectacular crash and burn episode on the ski fields at Lake Louise, Canada because 1) I didn't have the proper training and 2) I wanted to go fast and do stuff I wasn't prepared to do. (Quick extra note: don't succumb to a group of people telling you to "hurry up." It's a recipe for disaster!) My best advice participating in any sport is: *Slow down or stop before you lose complete control.* How many times have we neglected that little pearl to our own peril?

Another good approach is consulting a good quality fitness trainer if you're new to the physical activity thing. Now, on to the points at hand.

The What

'What' can be anything that requires you to move your body (preferably all of it), elevates the heart rate, causes you to sweat (great for detoxing the body), and pushes or pulls against some type of resistance. Let me go a little deeper into the basic principles of resistance.

Muscles only grow as a result of being pushed or pulled against something. It's like the body over-compensates when we lift something heavy, saying, "Damn, that was heavy! I think we better make more muscle fibers in case we have to lift that again." Our amazing body constantly evolves to deal with bigger and bigger challenges.

The brain works the same way. When it's challenged it grows. It becomes more resilient. It rewires itself to deal with greater challenges. How about that? Whether physical or mental, the challenges in life are just what we need to help us to grow and step into a greater field of possibility.

Now, movement options are endless and include most of the sports played around the world—football, soccer, tennis, volleyball, rowing, catch-and-kiss, cycling, swimming, etc. There are specific health and fitness activities like weight training, aerobics classes, dance, yoga, Pilates, martial arts, gymnastics, boxing, and more. There are activities combing mind and body like Qigong, Tai Chi, and yoga. Then there are adventure-type pursuits like running, hiking, mountain biking, climbing, skiing, trekking and many more. There is no shortage of things to choose from.

Bottom line, the 'what' comes down to the things you LIKE to do. It's no good signing up at the local gym knowing you're unlikely to attend. Find something you like and go from there.

That's the basic formula. Here are some categories to choose from:

1. **Resistance training**. The best example is weight training, but that's not the only form. Chin-ups or push-ups, working with elastic resistance bands— whatever challenges the muscles, causing them to grow. These activities also help from a brain perspective, a hormonal balancing perspective, a functional perspective (preventing injury), a weight loss perspective and for cardiovascular health.

2. **Aerobic training**. This means you're doing something that steps up your breathing and heart rate, moving oxygen around the cardiovascular system—and doing it longer than a few breaths! Step classes, pump classes, Zumba© classes, running, power walking, dancing, swimming, are all aerobic activities.

3. **Active Mind-Body training**. I use the word 'active' to differentiate this from the other mind-body practices like meditation. Optimum health means physical and mental health, and these are the kinds of activities that contribute to both. Yoga, Tai Chi, and Qigong and other forms of highly conscious martial arts fit into this category. Yoga has been around ever

since the Adi Yogi in India created it over 10,000 years ago. Qigong has been around for 4,000 years. The reason they're still around is because they WORK.

In the next chapter I'll go into more detail about the best combination of resistance, aerobic and active mind-body training. In the meantime, let's move on to the next 'W.'

The When

The best time to exercise is... drum roll please:

Whenever you're most likely to do it!

I often pray clients prefer the morning. (It's OK if you don't!) And the reason I pray it's a morning routine is:

1. It energizes you at the start of the day, making you more alert and cognitively functional, allowing you to better plan the day ahead. Remember, elite athletes set the tempo for a peak performance by warming up before the start of the game. If we want to be elite human beings, we need to set ourselves up at the start of our day so we have the highest probability of success.

2. It's the one time of day you can most control. You decide when to set your alarm clock. If you train in the afternoon, there are often competing priorities, which means you miss a training session.

3. Yoga was once a predominantly morning practice because tapping into the energy released with the rising sun's rays connects you to increasing energy and the cycles between the environment and your body's internal chemistry.

Though I encourage a morning start, any time of the day is great to exercise. I remember when I was doing weight training in my early 20's that afternoon workouts could be a drag to get started since I was tired after a long day at work. I also told myself I couldn't do weight training in the morning. Fast-forward to my 30s and suddenly I'm doing weight training in the mornings and it works just fine. In fact, it's more than just fine. I'm more focused, clear, resilient to stress, creative and productive. Try it yourself to see if you experience the same benefits.

The How Much

Now we're getting into murky waters. I'm not sure if you've heard of the F.I.T.T. Principle? It was designed to be a policy statement on exercise prescription for differing populations. The acronym stands for:

1. Frequency (F). How often you exercise per week.
2. Intensity (I). How hard you train. Can you still talk and train or are you sucking in breaths like your life depended on it?
3. Timing (T). How long you're recommended to train for each session and total per week.
4. Type (T). What types of exercises.

Standards have changed over time, and about the only thing national safety councils and heart foundations agree on now is the need for different types of exercises (resistance and aerobic) and the benefit of doing exercise at a high enough intensity to make it a physical challenge.

Everyone is different and most people are at different levels of fitness. As your optimum health coach, I work on the initial principle that 'any' is better than none. So if you're doing none, then five minutes a day of 'something' is a great start.

The first thing for people starting from scratch is getting into the habit of showing up. Three minutes of walking in place is super-duper. Got that covered? Then take it up to five minutes, then onwards and upwards until you get to a place and space that looks like the following:

1. **Frequency**. Four to six times per week—preferably six with a day of rest. Again, I want to stress this is about building up to this place.

2. **Intensity.** This comes in two parts. First, you need to mix up the intensity. Make some sessions hard. Do some on medium and some on the easy setting. The other thing is the intensity of movement needs to be enough to be an effort to perform. No effort = no growth = limited to zero benefit.

3. **Timing.** This can vary greatly depending on the level of intensity. Unless you're an athlete training for something specific, I rarely see the need to go over 60 minutes—unless, of course, the activity is hiking or walking or something of a lower intensity which you can sustain for a longer period of time.

4. **Type.** This is where I differ slightly from a lot of general fitness professionals. Like most, I suggest a mix of aerobic and resistance training. But I also recommend doing some Active Mind-Body Training as well. After all, we're talking about optimum health for the body and mind, so without this you miss out on amazing mental benefits.

Next chapter I'll guide you through my own personal activities regime just to give you an example—and more detailed information!

CHAPTER 9:

Physical Activity Carl Massy style

There is a saying about people sacrificing their health to create wealth and then spending their wealth trying to get their health back. A much better choice is to make conscious movement part of your general lifestyle throughout your life.

I've always been very active, partly because of good habits instilled by my father. To this day, at the prime young age of 72, he still gets up early (4 am-ish) to do a weights workout, then goes for a walk, then is likely to go for a bicycle ride during the day as well. The other reasons I'm active include vanity (luckily much less these days), my love of a challenge, the endorphin high, and the inner knowing my body needs it. Plus, it allows me to go on adventures — like a week hiking in Nepal, trekking the Inca trail, or cross country running through the snow in the Walls of Jerusalem mountain range in Tasmania.

Being active not only keeps us healthy longer, it gives us more options in life.

Reasons come first

The reason I started this chapter with all the reasons I stay active is because it's the reasons we have to do things and the emotions associated with those reasons that cause us to act. We talked about this in the introduction when I asked you why optimum health is a MUST for you. The more emotionally charged our reasons, the more physical energy and life force impetus we gain to do what needs to be done, the more successful we are.

Here are some more reasons why physical activity is a MUST for me:

1. I'll never have the energy, vitality or health to be able to express my full potential if I do not move my body daily.
2. My mind is much clearer and more creative when I exercise.
3. I have more energy to achieve a higher level of success.
4. I would be a complete phony and would feel like a total loser if I didn't maintain an awesome physical training regime,
5. I want to live a mentally and physically active life well into my 'twilight' years.

Given all my reasons, exercise is not a question of 'should I?' It's more: 'How could I not, knowing what's at stake?

My physical training regime

As a general guideline for you, this is what I do. Variety is the spice of life, and I like to mix things up. But there's a practical reason for it too. The body is very good at becoming efficient at doing the same thing over and over again, taking less energy to get the job done. If you want to burn the most calories and constantly challenge your body, create a variable routine.

For me, a typical week might look like this:

1. Monday – Beach run. 45-60 minutes. Medium intensity.
2. Tuesday – Yoga class. 60 minutes. Hard. Jelly legs.
3. Wednesday – Bike ride. 45 minutes. Easy - Medium.
4. Thursday – Weights at the gym or body weight workout. 20 minutes. Hard.
5. Friday – AM: Dance. 15-20 minutes. Fun. PM: Yoga. 90-minute class. Restorative yoga. Stretching deep muscles. Easy – Medium.
6. Saturday – Ride or beach run or a mix of stuff. 60 minutes. Medium.
7. Sunday – REST. Yippee!!

My training is more about results and return on investment then a social occasion—not that you can't blend both results and fun social experiences. Personally, I want the biggest return in the shortest possible time; a routine that challenges my body, burns energy, doesn't damage my body over the long term, is something I enjoy, requires the least amount of props and preparation, is interchangeable, and keeps me feeling and looking fit and healthy.

I'm not anal on ticking all of these boxes, but I definitely tick most, most of the time.

Obviously, this is ideal for *me*. You need to find your own swagger and routine. But whatever you choose, if you lean into doing movement with focused purpose and consciousness, you get better results and are least likely to hurt yourself.

All that said, remember, change is the essence of life. If I'm getting ready for a specific activity or adventure—like a tough mountain trek or week long river paddle, I may adjust the type and intensity of my training. Being too rigid with anything we do leads to inflexibility in our thinking and our bodies. As we get older we may need to amend and adjust how and what we do. (Stopping as you get older is NOT an option!) Having a big chest, six-pack abs and huge arms is not the major priority it was in my 20s. Even though I'm conscious of wanting to look good, nowadays my training priority is always about health, happiness, vitality and longevity. I rely more on my (obvious) wisdom, wit and charm to impress than my biceps!

In more detail

I want to go into a bit more detail about what I do, how I do it, and a bit more of the 'why' behind everything.

Monday

Running. Aerobic activity. 45-60 minutes.

I live in Bali, so I'd be a dingbat if I didn't get down to the beach on a regular basis. Before I go for a run, I meditate for at least 15 minutes. Listening to the sound of the ocean at the start of the day at the start of the week is a great way to kick things off. If you can, find somewhere special to start your week.

As I'm running on the sand, I let my mind wander. I gaze out over the water and just enjoy the experience of moving my body in the great outdoors. Running on sand is also great for strengthening the smaller muscles responsible for the stability of the ankles and knees. You just need to pay attention to where you're stepping. This session is probably about medium intensity. If I want to take it a little higher, I might add some running backwards or mini-sprints.

Tuesday
Yoga. Active Mind-Body. 60 minutes.

This is a relatively new addition to my program. I find I can push and motivate myself (and others) easily with training. But every now and again it's great to let someone else push me. Plus there's the added collective energy in a group session. This particular yoga class is taught by Octavio Salvado, an Australian instructor I've interviewed a number of times for *The Happiness Class* (iTunes Channel). It's a hard, inwardly focused workout. The postures are demanding and require a deep focus on where and what the body is doing. My legs are like jelly during and after the class.

Wednesday
Bike ride. Aerobic activity. 45 minutes.

Riding a bike is a great activity because it works out the legs and some of the biggest muscles in the body. You can also do a high intensity session on a bike and still not have any detrimental impact on the knee joints and ankles. Another great low impact exercise is swimming. Most of us (including me) don't have immediate access to a lap pool, so swimming requires more logistics and time than I like to spend. I also don't swim much because I'm pretty crap at swimming.

Thursday

Weights. Resistance training. 10-20 minutes.

In 2012 I read a book called *Body by Science* by McGuff (MD) and Little (top fitness researcher in USA). They wanted to find the most effective exercise regime for health, longevity, performance, etcetera for the least commitment of time. My kind of stuff, ROI (return on investment) focused! As a result I do a 10-15 minute weights workout once a week.

I won't go into detail here because you need some weight training experience or a good trainer to do this. But all the muscle fibers in the body need to be challenged at some point in the week. Doing a minimum of one resistance training session is essential for your health and body function—especially as you get older. And you don't need to use weights or go to a gym to do this.

Resistance training can also be done with your body weight, like push-ups, pull-ups, or dips and squats. Plus you don't need to train for an hour or more to get the benefits. Great results can be had in a focused 10-20 minute session. If time is short, I do a weight session at home including push-ups, dips, upside-down push-ups (definitely not for newbies), and pull-ups with a specially mounted bar at the entrance to my office. I just do as many reps as I possibly can in one set. I do push-ups until I cannot do one more. Then I move on to the next exercise. So it's a pretty quick session but great return on investment!

Friday

(AM) Dance. Aerobic activity and fun. 15 minutes.

I set my iPod up or play some funky tunes through YouTube and away I go. Total freestyle. No rules. No limitations, but a whole lot of fun.

When we're relaxed, moving, light of spirit and having fun, we can be extremely creative. I've also been known to use this activity to help with brainstorming. I'll dance in my office with a clean whiteboard in front of me. Any time I get an idea I write it down. This is called 'stream of consciousness' or getting in 'flow.'

(PM) Yoga. Active Mind-Body activity. 90 minute class.

You definitely need to do at least one activity each week that stretches out the muscles. A lot of the work we do contracts the muscles, so to balance that out we want to streeeeeeeetch (our body and mind).

My favorite activity for this is yoga—one of the life-changing practices I incorporated into my routine in 1999.

Yoga transformed my life because, not only did I do the physical activity, I studied the philosophy behind it. The true practice of Yoga has the ability to not only make you a more healthy person, but it can help you to become a much more self-aware and externally aware person.

My Friday afternoon class is designed to round out my week by releasing tension I may have built up working. It's a deep stretch class (Yin Yoga), where you hold what at first seems like gentle postures for up to 5 minutes each. But when you stay in one position more than a minute or two, the mind starts to wander and complain and you can experience some pain or discomfort.

This is a powerful internal tonic for both the body and the mind. Yoga rocks. And so does Angela Perez, our great Spanish yoga instructor.

Saturday
Riding. Aerobic activity. 45-60 minutes.

Generally there is more time on a Saturday, so I like to make this more of a fun day. (Though my idea of fun might be different from yours!) My idea of fun is a longer ride or a longer run. But to make it more fun I'm more selective of the location. For instance, I ride through more rice fields, or go for a run down the beach. This might be a good day to do activities with friends — like a great game of tennis, or squash, or football, etc.

The final word

This is just a general idea of what I might do in a week. I mix it up and lengthen or shorten things as required. I might also add or subtract things because I have a friend visiting who wants to do a particular type of activity. Or I might have an injury or ailment at times, so I have to mix it up. Recently I had a swollen knee as a result of doing a bunch of Jackie Chan moves without being warmed up (aka: being an idiot). So my daily physical activities are modified accordingly (as opposed to stopping).

Remember, movement is LIFE. (Which means the opposite is?) Once you stop moving the body, your health starts to move backwards. Your muscles atrophy rather quickly, and all the great benefits you were experiencing start taking a backseat.

Don't use limited time as an excuse to do nothing! If I only have 10 minutes I choose 10 activities that require no props and do one minute of each with no rest in between — like lunges, squats, star jumps, knee-raises, jumping on the spot, push-ups, etc. Be creative.

I also do energizing exercises 365 days of the year. They take 3 minutes and I do them immediately before I meditate. To see an example, just do a search on *YouTube* for '*Carl Massy Energization Exercises*.' Doing this daily activity means that, regardless of what happens in my day, I know I've moved my body at least once. Even though it was only for a few minutes it's better than no movement at all. Movement is not just good physically; it's good psychologically because I feel better about myself.

CHAPTER 10:

Weight Loss and Physical Activity

One of the biggest issues for many people is weight management and weight loss. Given the rapidly increasing number of people who are overweight or obese in developed and developing countries and the importance of maintaining a proportionate weight for optimal health, it definitely needs discussing.

Quite often you hear people say that weight loss is totally related to physical activity. But that's not the full story. I remember when my brother was competing in natural bodybuilding tournaments in Australia back in the 90's. He told me his success was about 30 percent due to his physical training and 70 percent due to nutritional management. He could work out less than someone else in the gym but look and be in much better shape because he understood and practiced better nutrition.

Getting physical without working on changing nutritional practices makes losing weight and improving your body's health a very slow process. The quickest way to lose weight is a combination of physical activity, nutrition, detoxification, changing your mindset and effectively processing emotional issues—essentially the 6 Pillars of this book.

So, here's a pop quiz. Which requires less effort and less time?
1. Forgoing a Starbucks double chocolate chip brownie
2. Going for a 5 mile (8km) run

If you eat the brownie, which is about 400 calories and takes less than 5 minutes to consume, you'll need to run for about 45 minutes to expend those calories. Yikes! Looked at that way it becomes VERY obvious if you want to make the biggest impact on weight loss that it's much more efficient to make better nutritional choices. Who has 45 minutes (which is often a 75-minute activity when you consider changing clothes, transit times, etc) to offset every 'bad' high-calorie food choice made?

Yes, movement is highly important for weight management for various reasons, including regulating your hunger. But without a conscious approach to nutrition and an understanding of the biggest nutritional villains, the weight loss game can be extremely challenging.

IF – THEN Strategy

So, what to do? That damn brownie keeps calling your name. How do you make the better choice? The first thing is to educate yourself, which you're doing with this book (especially in the next section on nutrition). The second thing is developing the ability to raise your consciousness in any given moment (which we'll address when we get to Mindfulness). The third thing to help you succeed (which is related to number two) is using what I call the IF-THEN Strategy.

First, figure out what situations and foods trigger you and what reactions those things elicit. Then replace the unconscious *reaction* with a *response* of your choosing. Here's an example:

IF I go to a social gathering and I'm offered an unhealthy snack, THEN I will politely decline and seek out a healthy option.

Based on the assumption you've educated yourself well enough to understand *unhealthy* and *healthy* choices, the reasons this strategy works is because:

1. Once you set the intention (IF this happens, THEN I'll do that) you are setting your mind up to look for opportunities to activate this strategy.
2. You do not need to use willpower when the unhealthy snack is offered because you've already made your choice. (Remember, using willpower expends a LOT of energy in the brain.)
3. Choosing a strategy makes you more conscious of the choices you have.

Other examples of effective IF-THEN strategies related to making better choices include:

- IF I am hungry, THEN I will not go grocery shopping.
- IF I am going to drink alcohol, THEN I will not drive.
- IF I meet a hot girl or guy that smokes, THEN I will not get involved with them romantically (I didn't know this strategy in the past, so I went through some serious heart-ache back in the day).
- IF it's Sunday, THEN I can eat a really crappy desert at lunchtime.
- IF I catch my new partner lying, THEN I will decide whether I want to be in this relationship.

When we make a choice in advance we're not under duress when the time comes to put it into action. We can be relaxed and thinking at our best as we implement our decision.

Here's an example of this strategy and how well it works. In 2001, after finishing my time with the Army, I traveled around the world for a year before starting a new job. About midway through the year I was at Tikal Ruins in Guatemala. Feeling totally blissed-out, I wrote down my ideal criteria for a new job when I got back to Australia. In it I included a couple of deal-breakers in the form of IF-THEN strategies. One was IF the work did not provide opportunities for international travel THEN I would turn it down.

When I got back, I got offered a great job (on paper). But it didn't offer the travel opportunities I'd decided were crucial. Much to the surprise of the potential employer, I turned it down. But then, as life does, I was offered another option—a contract to consult to the Salt Lake 2002 Winter Olympic Games, which ticked all my boxes.

My point is, trust your best thinking that comes when you're in a relaxed and highly conscious state of mind. Think about what IF-THEN strategies you'd like to incorporate into your life around fitness, health, food, relationships, business opportunities and the like. Set great IF-THEN strategies and honor them. Step in the direction you chose when you're at your best and you'll very likely create a life that's in alignment with your best.

One of the challenges

One of the biggest challenges with weight loss and physical activity is the fact that when we exercise, we're highly likely to feel hungrier. It'd be nice if the body would just tap our excess body fat stores to get its energy needs met, but our bodies aren't designed to work like that. Survival dictates that we store body fat for times of famine. So the body doesn't give up that excess body fat easily. Plus, if your body is insulin resistant, there are metabolic issues that impede the normal functioning of fat cells. I'll go into more detail about insulin issues when we talk about nutrition.

Evolution has made it so the body sends a signal after physical activity, telling us we need to eat. And it prompts us to go for a high-energy source (chocolate brownie here I come!). Therefore, if you're trying to lose weight, make sure before your workout that you've given thought to what you will *eat after your workout*. That way you can ensure you're putting the best fuel in your body. Also make sure you drink plenty of water after working out, as this will also help suppress your hunger.

I go into more details in the section on nutrition, but the best food choices after a workout are high in nutrients, high in fiber, with good quality protein and fat and not processed. An example might be a big salad with plenty of nuts and seeds for that extra protein and quality fats, or a wrap with similar ingredients or a piece of fruit with a handful of raw nuts.

If you want to lose weight, **never work out without considering what you are going to eat and drink after you have finished.**

CHAPTER 11:

The Practice of Yoga

I'm a big fan of a physical practice that ticks all of the physical activity boxes while maintaining a holistic approach to health and wellbeing—and that's yoga. Here's a summary of the five biggest benefits by yoga instructor and wellness teacher Octavio Salvado who is the co-founder of *The Practice* in Bali.

5 Benefits of Practicing Yoga by Octavio Salvado

In the practice of yoga there is no such thing as absolute stillness. Our biology is a comprehensive system designed to move in a skillful yet organic way, and every part of our being, down to the smallest cell, is in a state of constant balanced movement. In ancient times yoga was referred to as 'Skill in Action,' because it invites practitioners not to simply participate in life, but to participate with precision and move with purpose. When we do this, our entire mind/body system benefits greatly.

BENEFIT 1 - Vitality

In yoga there is a concept known as 'Bramha Grunthi,' which is one of the 'knots' restricting us from reaching our highest personal potential. This particular knot deals with inertia. Through lack of movement, energy becomes lodged in the physical components of our being, like the muscles, tendons, ligaments and joints, creating a solidifying effect we call stiffness. Through skillful movement, as in the actions of Hatha Yoga, some of this energy is released as the muscles and tendons are elongated, resulting in a liberation of energy we feel as vitality.

BENEFIT 2 - Wellbeing

Once liberated through mindful movement (particularly when the movement is accompanied by conscious breathing), the now freely flowing energy enters the nervous system, moving back towards the command center of the brain, causing a release of various hormones and neuropeptides which result in a feeling of well-being and emotional happiness. Conversely, in the absence of movement, stiffness quickly leads to energetic blockages, creating states of fatigue, which, if prolonged, can result in depression. Fortunately, this is easily reversible with the practice of yoga.

BENEFIT 3 - Relaxation/Stress release

One of the major obstacles we face in terms of balancing our bodies and minds and achieving optimal, whole-system health is the over-stimulation of our nervous system. What we see, read, hear, think and in any way perceive through the senses, travels into the nervous system as vibration similar to traffic moving along a highway. The reason so many people today feel stressed and overwhelmed is because there's too much sensory traffic. Your system is jammed! There's too much information, too much stimulation. Yet the remedy is simple: Move and breathe. Movement liberates stuck energy. This is why people leave yoga classes more relaxed than when they came in.

BENEFIT 4 - Mindfulness

As the body becomes more vital and healthy, and excess charge is released from the nervous system, the energy flowing through it creates a feeling of wellbeing and peacefulness. This slowing down and recalibration aids whole-system balance, preparing the platform for mindfulness practices such as meditation. Without skillful action leading to the liberation of stuck energy, calmer states of being, a stronger and more flexible body and a meditative mind will remain elusive.

BENEFIT 5 - Confidence

Yoga connects us to our raw physicality — our muscles and bones and ligaments. And yet, if we develop the sensitivity through increased mindfulness, it can take us deeper. When we connect more consciously with our physical nature through movement, we begin to perceive more in terms of sensations coming from our bodies. Movements that once caused a feeling of resistance and pain become exhilarating experiences! It feels good to move! We greet opportunities with enthusiasm rather than struggle. As we deepen our practices and become more comfortable in our physical bodies, a healthy self-image is cultivated and confidence becomes our natural state of being. We feel adequate and capable and a sense of happiness about being active and successful in what we are doing develops.

CHAPTER 12:

Pillar 1 (Physical Activity) Summary

For this Pillar and for all of the summaries to come, I will highlight the key points and list specific Optimum Health Strategies I highly recommend you take. There will also be a list of resources if you want a deeper dive into the science and research behind my observations and suggestions.

When it comes to Physical Activity, these are the most important points:

1. Movement is essential to optimum health. You will never fulfil your true potential if you do not include different forms of focused and intentional movement into your lifestyle.
2. Movement is essential for maintaining optimal functioning of the immune and lymphatic systems.
3. Movement is essential in helping process excessive cortisol and adrenaline running havoc in most of our bodies as a result of the stress response.
4. Movement is essential for optimum functioning of the brain. It increases cognitive functioning, contributes to stress management and resilience, and is essential for neurogenesis.

Optimum Health Strategies

1. The body responds best to physical change. Mix up the activities you choose.
2. Include aerobic activities, resistance training, stretching and active Mind-

Body sessions. Include some easy, hard, medium, fun, and social sessions into your week.

3. Attend a local yoga class. This may very well be a major life-changer. It was for me!

4. Move 6 days a week. But build up to it if you are starting from scratch. Make it easy to succeed by including sessions like a brisk walk, or 100 star jumps on the spot, or cutting some funky dance moves for 15 minutes.

5. Schedule the sessions in your calendar or diary at the start of the week, noting exactly what you will do and when. As Winston Churchill said, "He who fails to plan, is planning to fail."

6. If you are unsure of how to construct and conduct a physical training routine, speak to a competent fitness professional. Make sure you find the right trainer for you with the right knowledge, mindset, enthusiasm and dedication to your results. The investment in your health will have a high Return on Investment (ROI).

Recommended Resources

Octavio Salvado is one of those unique yoga instructors and teachers who bring an amazing level of depth to his teachings and classes from a physical, emotional and mental perspective. If you ever come to Bali, join him at *The Practice* for an amazing session, or you can connect with Octavio through his website at: **www.octaviosalvado.com**

Books:

- *Spark* by Eric Hagerman and Dr. John Ratey
- *Finding Ultra* by Rich Roll
- *Modern Yoga* by Duncan Peak
- *Body by Science* by John Little and Doug McGuff
- *Born to Run* by Christopher McDougall
- *Autobiography of a Yogi* by Paramahansa Yogananda

Equipment:

Buy a set of hand weights to use at home if time is short or you can't access a fitness center. I have a few different sizes to choose from for different exercises. I have 2.2 pound (1kg), 4.4 pounds (2 kg) and 13.2 pounds (6 kg). Also a set of resistance exercise rubber bands from a fitness store is great if you're travelling or space is tight.

Free Stuff

Click on the Resources Tab at **www.theguidetooptimumhealth.com** to get:

- 10 simple exercises to create a 10-minute workout with no props
- Free eBook *50 Most Awesome Outdoor Exercises*

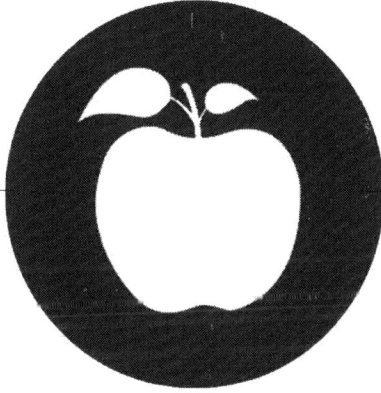

PILLAR 2
NUTRIENT ABUNDANCE

The doctor of the future will no longer treat the human frame with drugs, but rather will cure and prevent disease with nutrition.
Thomas Edison, American inventor and businessman

CHAPTER 13:

We really are what we eat

Nutrition is a major passion of mine. I devour (pardon the pun) books on nutrition like a teenager reads the Twilight Saga. For the last decade I've uncovered so much fascinating information I hardly know where to start. With the cavemen? Nomadic tribes? Agrarian societies? The amoeba? Okay, maybe I should spare you the history of the world food story and keep it practical. So, let's start with....

D - I - E - T

A little 4-letter word that is actually not bad in and of itself, the Oxford Online Dictionary lists two separate meanings for 'diet:'

1. The kinds of food that a person, animal, or community habitually eats; and

2. A special course of food to which a person restricts themselves, either to lose weight or for medical reasons.

We're going to stick with meaning #1 during our time because restrictions don't work. Most often the application of restrictions produces a result that is 180 degrees opposite from the original intention. The restriction of alcohol during American Prohibition from 1920–1933 was hardly a raging success — unless, of course, your name was Al Capone. How many times have we all sworn off sugar or some other 'bad' substance and ended up indulging even more in the end?

Whatever we place our attention upon is magnified. So the things we are restricting grow in importance and presence in our minds. It's like being told to stop thinking about a pink elephant. What do you end up thinking about? Exactly.

So here's the plan: we want to spend our time focused on what we DO want — the best nutrients to put into our bodies so we fill them with goodness and simply crowd out the crappy stuff. If we put 80 percent goodness into our bodies, there's only 20 percent space left to fit in the average or bad.

A nutritious diet is less about counting calories and more about the quality of the choices you make. Some of the most nutrient dense foods on Earth also happen to have the least amount of calories. Dr. Joel Fuhrman, the author of *Eat to Live* and *Super Immunity*, is a family physician, best-selling author and nutritional researcher specializing in nutritional healing. Dr. Fuhrman's very astute formula is $H = N / C$. In other words, Health (H) is directly proportional to the amount of Nutrients (N) we get for the amount of Calories (C) we consume.

In developed nations we've got this formula backwards. There's usually an excess of calories and a shortage of nutrients in our food due to over-processing and the prevalence of sugar and high fructose corn syrup (from genetically modified corn sources) in most products.

Following Furhman's advice (and mine!), if we fill up on the really good stuff (the healing foods), we get an enormous amount of nutrients into our bodies for a very small amount of calories. I know you're excited about that!

Optimum Health = Optimum Nutrients

In the nutrition game, optimum health is less about the proportions of *macronutrients* (protein, fat, carbohydrates) you consume and more about the amount of *micronutrients* you get into your body. By this I mean:

- Vitamins
- Minerals
- Fiber
- Phytonutrients

Vitamins and Minerals

We need essential vitamins and minerals on a daily basis. They're called 'essential' because our bodies can't manufacture them internally and we need to ingest them. There are 13 essential vitamins and over 30 minerals classified as macrominerals (e.g. calcium, chlorine, sodium, potassium, phosphorus, and magnesium) and trace minerals (e.g. chromium, zinc, manganese, copper, and iron). The trace minerals are called that because the body requires them in trace levels only.

If our diet is lacking in key vitamins and minerals our health will be affected both at the physical and mental level. It may not happen immediately because our bodies have amazing adaptive and protective abilities. But you will not be at your optimum without a *balanced* diet that facilitates the intake of these nutrients.

A quick note on vitamin D. Vitamin D is important because it promotes the absorption of calcium into the body, which is obviously essential for good bone health and other functions, like regulating the heart. Vitamin D exists in a number of animal products (fish, meat and eggs) and different mushrooms. However, the best (and free) source of vitamin D remains the sun. Just 20-minutes exposure to the ultra-violet rays of the sun and you're good to go on your vitamin D requirements for the day.

Fiber

Optimum health not only requires good nutrients coming in, but it requires the effective removal of waste products via the bowels. We'll talk more about elimination when we get to the section on detoxification. But for now, know that we cannot be at our best health if we do not have a highly functional elimination system.

Fiber is *absolutely essential* for effective elimination of waste from our bowels and it only comes from plant sources (e.g. fruit, vegetables, nuts, seeds, and grains). If you aren't regular in your elimination, or not doing it with ease, then it's time to get more fiber into your diet (plus plenty of water of the natural non-chlorinated variety).

A great micronutrient source, fiber slows down the absorption of glucose into the bloodstream, keeping insulin levels steady. It also keeps fructose from overloading the liver. In addition, fiber helps alert the brain when we're full. So it plays a key role in our health. And yet, it's one of the micronutrients most under threat in the modern diet today.

Phytonutrients
Also referred to as phytochemicals, these are the chemicals that help plants defend against environmental challenges, such as disease, injury, pollutants, pests and ultraviolet light. There are about 10,000 phytochemicals and they only exist in plant sources. It's likely that phytonutrients protect us humans from many of the same things as well (maybe not the pests). But the scientific community is having a hard time definitively proving this.

Food in its natural state, picked from a tree, pulled out of the ground or harvested, has healing and health properties far beyond our modern scientific understanding. Plant medicine is as ancient as humanity. Hippocrates apparently used willow tree leaves to lower fevers. Native Americans used willow bark concoctions to relieve fever, pain and inflammation. And guess what? Salicin, which comes from the bark of the white willow tree, is what inspired the synthesis of its pharmaceutical counterpart, Aspirin.

There is an amazing symbiotic relationship between all plants and animals on this Earth. For me, a big part of our nutritional health comes down to tapping into these natural wonders.

Essential Fatty Acids

Essential fatty acids (EFAs) were originally called Vitamin F when they were first discovered. They now sit in the category of fats, but they actually work more like a micronutrient. The two EFA's are omega-3 and omega-6. Some of the sources for them are fish, flaxseeds, chia seeds, hemp oil, leafy green vegetables, walnuts, and sunflower seeds.

In the next chapter we'll get into macronutrients—fats, carbs and protein.

CHAPTER 14:

Macronutrients: Fat, Carbohydrate and Protein

This is generally where the whole nutrition scene gets confusing.

Everyone has a different opinion on how much of each macronutrient is optimum. But optimum for what? Obviously we're not interested in the nutritional regime for an elite athlete (which may not be a long-term healthy eating plan). And we're not interested in bulking up for a bodybuilding competition. We're all about optimum health, vitality, happiness and longevity. In line with this orientation, in this chapter I'm simply going to talk enough about the big three—fat, carbohydrate, and protein—so we have a common frame of reference while I try to reduce the conflicting advice from the armchair experts.

Remember, the point of this journey is not about being perfect. It's about being and feeling GREAT. As you will see, there's a lot of flexibility in the diet game. More than anything else, feeling great is about making BETTER choices.

Protein

Protein is an essential macronutrient. Some (not all!) of the essential roles of protein in the body are:

1. Structural support: collagen, hair, crystallins (eyes)

2. Enzymatic: catalyzing biochemical reactions
3. Hormonal: carrying messages between cells

Protein is made up of amino acids, which are referred to as essential and non-essential amino acids. Non-essential amino acids can be produced in the body if the essential amino acids are present. So we definitely need sources for the essential amino acids.

Here is where the mud-slinging usually starts about the best sources of protein and how much you need in your diet. So let me keep this simple. Protein exists in almost all foods, whether animal products or plant products. Protein exists (dare I say it?) in a donut. But before you take up donuts as your protein source let me add that the percentage of protein in a donut is minimal and sugar is prolific. Remember Dr. Fuhrman's formula? **H (health) = N (nutrition)/ C (calories).** Donuts are definitely in the red zone when it comes to nutrition!

The World Health Organization (WHO) recommends that 5 percent of calories should come from protein. Interestingly, mothers' milk, which is the ideal food source for the biggest growth spurt a human ever experiences (a baby grows twice its size in the first two years) is about 5 percent protein. However, WHO's 5 percent figure is low compared to many other sources.

For example, the Center for Disease Control (CDC) in the US recommends that 10 to 35 percent of daily calories come from protein. In my humble opinion and from my research, I firmly believe this and most other 'optimal protein' figures quoted in the dietary field are inflated to benefit the multi-billion dollar industries producing the biggest marketed protein sources—meat, dairy, poultry, protein bars, protein powders, etcetera. When big money is at stake the 'facts' can suddenly become a little grey.

The fact is, our protein needs can be solely supplied by either animal sources or plant sources. The idea that vegetarians can't meet all their protein needs is simply not true. As medical practitioner and nutritionist Dr. John McDougall points out in his April 2007 Newsletter: "Since plants are made up of structurally sound cells with enzymes and hormones, they are by nature rich sources of proteins. In fact, so rich are plants that they can meet the protein needs of the earth's largest animals: elephants, hippopotamuses, giraffes, and cows. You would be correct to deduce that the protein needs of relatively small humans can easily be met by plants."

People in different cultures have thrived without animal products being a part of their diet for 1000's of years. Where your protein comes from and how much of your calorie intake it constitutes is less important than what's packaged with that protein. Does it come with lots of micronutrients and fiber? Or does that yummy tin of sweet and sour Szechuan beef come with high sugar content or artificially produced trans fats that are toxic for the body? For me, the packaging is the bigger and better question.

Regardless of whether you're a meat-eater, vegetarian or vegan, you can get adequate protein from your own chosen diet. For optimum health, it's more about being aware what you're taking in (or not taking in) with the protein source and making the wise choice.

My final word on protein is the use of the word 'protein.' We need to get out of the incorrect idea of labeling some foods as protein and others not—as so many chefs do on the numerous cooking shows playing on television. Food sources have a combination of protein, carbohydrate, and fat as opposed to 100 percent of a single macronutrient. By calling a food a protein it wrongly projects the message that everything else not called a protein does not contain protein—which couldn't be farther from the truth. This is not educating people. It's misleading them, making people worry they will experience a protein deficiency because they're only eating beans, corn, vegetables and seeds, when all of these foods contain protein. So be conscious of the labels you use with the food you eat.

Carbohydrates

Carbohydrate is another grossly misunderstood word that gets thrown about by supposed experts. Carbohydrates are essentially sugar molecules, which are the preferred fuel source for the body and brain. They come in different forms, including glucose, fructose, sucrose, lactose (from milk) and are an essential part of our health, energy and healthy brain function.

When people talk about 'carbs' being bad for you they're missing the point. The problem is not with carbohydrates, which are essential. Again, it's about the packaging.

There are two very different forms of carbohydrate which I will over-simplify to make a point. There are complex carbohydrates (the good guys), which are formed by long, complex chains of sugar molecules. And there are simple carbohydrates (the bad guys or junk food), which are formed from simply one or two sugar molecules. Complex carbohydrates are dietary starches that include most fruits, vegetables, whole grains, legumes and seeds. Simple carbohydrates are sugars and include refined sugar, brown sugar, honey, maple syrup, molasses and corn syrup. Hello pastries, cakes, cookies, candies, donuts, white breads, sodas, etc. Simple carbohydrates have no fiber and no nutrients and play absolute havoc on the insulin regulation of the body.

I'll go into more detail on insulin and insulin resistance later. But for now know that excessive quantities of glucose or fructose (the two main offenders) cause insulin levels to spike. This puts extra strain on the liver. If repeated frequently, this can lead to a condition where the cells fail to respond to the normal functions of the insulin hormone, affecting energy regulation, fat storage and the transportation of amino acids throughout the body.

In the last 30 years an enormous industry has been created around the production of foods (and I use that term loosely) that are extremely low in nutrients but very high in sugar or fructose. The end result of eating these highly processed "foods" is poor health, obesity, diabetes and other related illnesses. It's an easy process to track. Just observe the health statistics in developed nations. Observe the health curve in underdeveloped nations as Western processed foods become available and popular. Native populations rapidly decline in health and longevity. We will look more closely at sugar and fructose and their impact on global health later in the Guide.

Fat

Fat is not your enemy. The right fats are your friends.

The human brain consists of about 60 percent fat. It's an essential macronutrient that transports nutrients around the body. Fat is also the most effective fuel source because there are 9 kilojoules of energy per gram of fat compared to carbohydrate, which is only 4 kilojoules per gram. Which is why the body stores fat as a reserve against hard times when the local antelope herd has migrated and all the berries have been picked off the bushes. All those excess calories stored as fat can be easily converted to energy by the body in hard times when food is scarce.

Given the vast time it takes for major evolutionary changes to occur in the metabolic functioning of the human body, we are still wired to seek out and hang onto the best fuel sources — fat. So it's important to know which kinds are best. Essentially there are four different types of fat:
1. Monounsaturated fats (good)
2. Polyunsaturated fats (good)
3. Saturated fats (some not quite as bad as we have been lead to believe)
4. Trans fats (artificially made and a total disaster for the body)

Monounsaturated fats are from plant sources (e.g. olives, avocado, nuts and seeds) and are, in my opinion, the best. Polyunsaturated fats are mostly from plant sources (e.g. nuts and seeds) and some fatty fish (e.g. salmon and trout) and are also a fine part of an optimum health diet.

Now we get to saturated fats and the fun begins.

There has been a 60-year campaign against saturated animal and dairy fats. We've been told that all saturated fat is bad for us because it increases the LDL cholesterol—the bad cholesterol. HDL is the good guy. But recent research suggests that while reducing saturated fats may reduce LDL, it does not necessarily correlate to lower risk of heart disease. Plus, not all saturated fats are created equal—keyword being "created." Trans fats are fats that have been artificially manipulated into a saturated state. Not only do trans fats increase LDL cholesterol, it's now been found that they *decrease* HDL in the body.

On the other hand, coconut oil is a saturated fat (along with palm oil and palm kernel oil) that has been used forever in Pacific Island populations where as much as 60 percent of total calorie intake may be from coconut oil. And yet all studies show their cholesterol levels and rates of cardiovascular disease are extremely low.

Again, it's important to look at the source. Plant-based saturated fats are a whole different animal from saturated fats in meats and dairy, let alone manufactured trans fats.

For optimum health, you want to avoid trans fats like you would an ex-partner on the psycho side. Trans fats are sneakily (and unethically) added to a lot of processed foods under the guise of *hydrogenated* or *partially hydrogenated* oils in order to increase the shelf life of products (and the profit margins). About 80 percent of trans fats are added to food and 20 percent are naturally occurring in meat and dairy products. The Australian Heart Foundation not only lobbied to have trans fats listed on food labels, but are also lobbying to have artificial trans fats banned as a food additive.

Bottom line? The best way to avoid trans fat on the path to optimum health is to consume more natural whole foods, eat less processed foods and read the labels on the processed foods you do eat. And don't be afraid of the good fats!

Remember, your brain is made of 60 percent fat. Perhaps there might be some correlation between the shocking rise in mental disorders and Alzheimer's Disease in the last 60 years and the whole "no fat" approach to diet?

And here's something else to get you thinking. Turns out the 'war on fat' was based on wrong and incomplete information. Fat doesn't make you fat — sugar does. I'll be going into a lot more detail on refined sugar and fructose shortly. But for now I just wanted to let fat off the hook. It's an essential macronutrient for optimum health. Refined sugar, on the other hand, is another (more sinister) story.

CHAPTER 15:

It's all about making better choices

When it comes to nutrition (as with any other subject) the ideal is not about being *extreme*. It's not about being rigid. It's not about being an evangelist for your nutritional beliefs. It's about adopting the best of the best. It's about listening to your own body's needs and modifying your diet as required. Maybe you're aiming to lose weight, or gain weight, or train for a marathon, or recover from an injury or illness. You may have to modify the foods you eat or lean a little bit more in one direction for a time.

To help you make better food choices, I've created a simple checklist as well as a visual image divided into zones which will give a basic idea about where food might sit on a spectrum from 'danger' to 'healing.' First the checklist.

The Optimum Nutrition Checklist

When it comes to diet, nutrition and optimum health there are a few general principles which essentially form a checklist split into the OPTIMUM and the UNHEALTHY camps of nutrition.

The OPTIMUM

- Produced by Mother Nature (she's still number one)

- Eaten in its original whole-food form (not processed)

- Freshly picked or harvested (in season)

- Organic (free from pesticides, herbicides, chemical fertilizers, and artificial processing)

- Locally produced (reducing the need for artificial storage and excessive transportation)

- Water-rich (our bodies are over 70% water)

- High in micronutrients (vitamins, minerals, protective enzymes, probiotics)

- High in phytonutrients (protective health benefits)

- High in dietary fiber

The UNHEATHY

- Highly processed (doesn't resemble the original food)

- Artificially flavored, colored, preserved, and manipulated

- Contains or is cooked with trans fat

- High calorie value but very low nutrient value

- Added sugar or fructose (contributes to insulin resistance)

- Contains MSG (monosodium glutamate)

- Contains artificial sweeteners (Aspartame, Acesulfame potassium, Saccharin, Sucralose)

- Known to contain toxic substances like heavy metals

Using this simple checklist you can look at most foods and have the ability to make an informed choice. Obviously, the aim is to tick as many boxes in the Optimum list and as few (or no) boxes in the Unhealthy list as possible.

Next we'll look at the different zones on a spectrum from healthy (optimum) to dangerous (unhealthy) when it comes to nutrition.

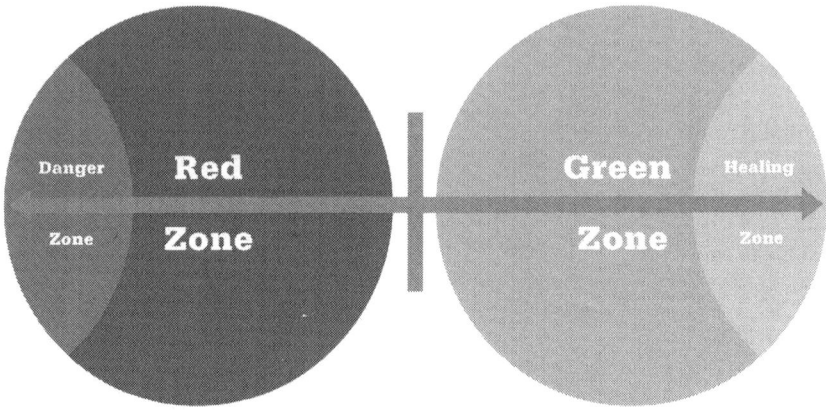

The Healing Zone
All ticks in The Optimum. No ticks in The Unhealthy.

This is the healing zone. You're selecting all the Optimum food choices. But you can up the ante in this zone by focusing on eating the 'superfoods' which are mainly your dark green leafy vegetables. Dr. Joel Fuhrman, author of *Super Immunity*, lists kale, watercress, collard greens, mustard greens, turnip greens, Bok Choy, and spinach at the top of his list of superfoods. Each of these is extremely high in immune boosting nutrients and fiber, but very low in calories. By eating a lot of these foods you're actually extending your life, preventing disease, and healing yourself from any illnesses you might have.

The Green Zone
Most ticks in The Optimum. A few ticks in The Unhealthy.
You eat some superfoods. You're enjoying organic vegetables, legumes and

fruits—broccoli, carrots, cabbage, lentils, peas, beans, peanuts, mangoes, bananas etcetera. And, of course, we all know you'd have to eat a bucket of kale leaves to feel, if not satisfied, then at least not hungry. This it is not about becoming a rabbit. Variety is the spice of life. Speaking of which, don't forget spices—turmeric, ginger, coriander, and cinnamon just to name a few.

These foods may not be dubbed as 'superfoods' but they're great for optimum health and may actually constitute a large part of your diet. Maybe you can't always find or afford organic local produce. Be sure to wash those non-organic fruits and veggies well! And the occasional ice cream cone or brownie? Well, it's not optimum, but it's important to enjoy the eating experience. The best way to do that is to mix it up when it comes to flavors and ingredients. Just make sure the majority are nourishing and replenishing for the body.

The Red Zone
Most ticks in The Unhealthy. A few ticks in The Optimum.

Most of your food comes heavily packaged and processed: Spicy Batter Fried Chicken Nuggets, Ranch Flavored Nacho Chips, Szechuan Noodles with Vegetables in Sweet and Sour Sauce with a few steamed veggies on the side to ease the guilt. You live in a world of highly processed foods, with high relative quantities of sugar and sugar substitutes like high fructose corn syrup, high levels of processed salt and very little existing nutrients. Only those vegetables (snap frozen or a whole food without additives in a can) and the occasional salad make it into the green zone.

The Danger Zone
All ticks in The Unhealthy. No ticks in The Optimum.

You already know where you are!

The unfortunate thing about food is that we figure if it's being sold in the supermarket it must be safe for our bodies. But even when a food is said to be safe that doesn't mean it's any good for us. Remember, once upon a time smoking was recommended as good for helping us relax!

If you're in this zone, now you know what you're doing to your body and you have the knowledge to make different choices. Take it step by step, but set the intention to get yourself into the green zone. In the meantime, the real baddies to look out for are foods containing:

- Trans fat – artificially made fat.

- MSG (Monosodium Glutamate) – this is a flavor enhancer used in lab rats to fatten them to obesity and it comes under a variety of chemical names. It is highly suspect.

- Artificial (synthetic) sweeteners. This is a highly debated topic and also a multi billion-dollar industry, so it's pretty difficult to get consistent or reliable facts on the health impact of artificial sweeteners. My preference is to avoid artificial sweeteners in general.

- Excessive added refined sugar or fructose.

The Grey Zone

I learned a long time ago that life is not all black and white. When I was living in Greece I was in a relationship and my girlfriend was Greek. Typical for the culture she resided most of the time in the 'grey zone.' In the grey zone you can still smoke a cigarette every now and again and, when asked about smoking, be adamant you're a non-smoker. For someone in the black or white zone, one puff on one cigarette automatically qualifies someone as a smoker. I used to hang out in the black or white zone. These days, with more wisdom under my belt, I like to be more like that willow in the wind that bends a bit.

So many things in life are hard to put into a specific box where you can say this applies 100 percent of the time in 100 percent of cases. The only time that's true is for universal laws like gravity. Otherwise there are always likely to be exceptions. The grey zone is something that leans more towards the green zone or more towards the red zone depending on other factors. In fact, as you can see in the diagram below, it may overlap both the green and the red zone.

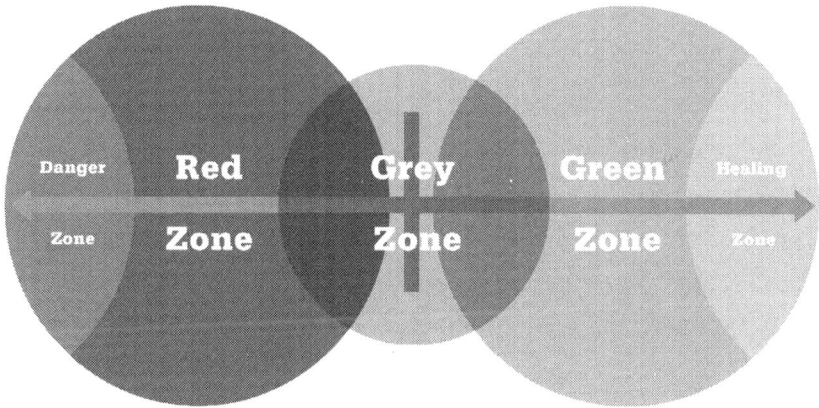

One of the best examples I can give for foods that are in the grey zone, oscillating between the green and red zones, are many animal products. Let's look at chicken. Which end of the Grey Zone do you think chicken would be if it was factory-farmed, traumatized, injected with antibiotics and hormones to make it grow faster, force fed, bathed 24/7 with artificial lighting, and unceremoniously handled, slaughtered and packaged for the supermarkets? If you haven't seen this process, I suggest you check out the highly informative DVD *Food Inc*.

On the other hand, which end of the Grey Zone does chicken reside if it's been locally raised in an open pasture, able to freely roam and forage, getting adequate sunlight, free from pesticides, hormone treatment and antibiotics, and then humanely slaughtered, packaged and sold locally? Which is better to bring inside your precious body? Which do you think would provide you higher levels of health and nourishment?

There is an equally significant difference between a locally grown organic apple and the apples in a mass-produced supermarket apple pie, which most likely has been sprayed with pesticides and herbicides, picked early, frozen, transported great distances and artificially ripened. Again, it's about making better choices with what's available to you—which might mean occasionally choosing to go without.

The other time a food source can go from Optimum to Unhealthy is when it's consumed in excess. Our bodies require a broad range of foods to ensure we get all the necessary nutrients for optimum health. If we overeat apples, for example, scoffing ten a day, regardless that they're a great food, they start to become less effective and potentially upset our internal digestive system.

CHAPTER 16:

Need to Know Nutritional Information

We touched on some of this information in the last chapter. Now it's time to go deeper. Nutrition is complex, so it's easier taking it in small bites!

Simple Carbohydrates, hormonal imbalances and weight gain

I can sum this whole subject up in one sentence: Even at very low levels, refined sugar and processed fructose are toxic to the body. And I'm not the only one saying that. Along with countless other health professionals, Dr Robert Lustig, author of *Fat Chance: The Truth About Sugar, Obesity and Disease*, calls sugar (and fructose) a toxin. Gary Taubes, in his book *Why We Get Fat*, says, "The very worst foods for us, almost assuredly, are indeed sugars—sucrose (table sugar) and high-fructose corn syrup in particular."

In *The Cholesterol Myth*, authors Jonny Bowden and Stephen Sinatra suggest plaque formation on the walls of blood vessels that cause blockages is likely initiated by oxidation from excessive sugar (or glucose) in the bloodstream—not fat. The oxidation causes ruptures in the blood vessels that set the process for plaque build-up in motion.

Decades ago, when food companies went down the low-fat path, they removed fat from food, which made their products less palatable. The solution was to add more sugar. Today, about 80 percent of processed foods on the market have refined sugars as ingredients, all of which are linked to insulin resistance, Metabolic Syndrome, obesity, Type II Diabetes and other major diseases. If we put sugar up against Dr. Fuhrman's H = N (nutrition) / C (calories) formula, it fails miserably. When it comes to a contest between sugars and fat for the worst possible food substance, the winner is sugar by a landslide. And the evidence just keeps mounting.

The World Health Organization suggests people greatly reduce their consumption of sugar due to potentially harmful effects and health consequences. It also recently reduced the recommended amount of calories derived from sugar on a daily basis from 10 percent to 5 percent. This equals about 25 grams or about six teaspoons of sugar for someone on a 2000-calorie diet. To put this in perspective, just one 12-ounce can of Coca Cola has 39 grams of refined sugar. Add that to all the rest of the sugar in most peoples' food and it's no wonder we have an obesity epidemic.

The effects of sugar on the body
Insulin
When sugar enters the body without fiber, it is quickly processed in the stomach to become glucose and then enters the bloodstream. The pancreas secretes the hormone insulin to regulate how the body's cells use and store glucose and fat. Insulin also allows the glucose from the blood to be stored in the liver and muscles as glycogen. If there is excess glucose in the blood, insulin converts this to saturated body fat.

If you consume a diet high in sugar, the body continues to produce more and more insulin until the body's cells and tissues no longer respond effectively to insulin (which is essentially insulin resistance and Type II Diabetes). At the cellular level it means ineffective management and storage of energy. Also, when insulin levels are elevated, we accumulate a variety of fat called triglycerides that take up a more permanent residence in our fat tissues. Unfortunately, triglycerides are unlikely to be released until insulin levels drop significantly. Over time, the excessive demands on the pancreas to produce insulin can also lead to a loss of insulin producing cells. Excessive insulin and the resultant insulin resistance also has a knock-on impact on other hormonal and metabolic functions, effectively taking the body out of homeostasis (balance).

The brain and stomach dialogue

When we eat a steady diet of highly processed foods with high amounts of added sugar and very low fiber levels, we're eating something foreign. Really. Our bodies weren't designed to process Boston Cream Pie. Our bodies are actually wired to think sweet foods, like bananas and berries are 'safe' foods, as opposed to bitter flavors, which indicate something poisonous. So the body naturally is inclined to want more of whatever tastes sweet. Plus, sweet things taste good! But there's a biochemical reason it's hard to stop eating sweets or drinking sweet beverages as well. Without fiber along with the sugar, the digestive system is less effective signaling the brain to stop eating.

In addition, the hypothalamus (which is at the base of the brain) controls energy balance and many of the hormonal systems within the body, including one of the hormones linked to insulin levels. Leptin is a master hormone that controls hunger and feelings of satiety. When there is Leptin resistance, which is common in most overweight and obese people, the brain almost goes into starvation mode thinking there is a shortage of food.

In his book *Fat Chance*, Dr. Lustig says, "When the brain can't see the leptin signal, it interprets starvation. The vagus nerve goes into overdrive to store more energy, and kick-starts the pancreas to make extra insulin - even more than the glucose rise would predict. This excess insulin release drives nonstop energy storage [as fat] and nonstop weight gain."

In other words, the brain mistakenly thinks the body is starving and signals that it wants more carbohydrate-rich food. It wants more energy stored in fat tissues and it wants less movement to conserve the energy that it mistakenly thinks it does not have. That is a pretty serious chain of events, definitely not leading to optimum health.

Addiction

According to research by Bartley Hoebel of Princeton University, sugar (or fructose) triggers a response in the same part of the brain that is targeted by cocaine, alcohol, nicotine, and other addictive substances known as the 'reward center.'

Could this get any worse? It might be that people are fixated on 'foods' that are high in sugar and an overconsumption of these foods because they are biochemically addicted to sugar in a way that causes them to behave with limited control or awareness. It's all happening at an internal biological level that's invisible to them.

My recommendation

Again, eat whole foods. Significantly reduce processed foods, especially the ones with very little fiber. The good news is, whole foods purchased in bulk or from a local farmers market are often less expensive than the highly processed excessively packaged refined 'foods' that are making the world sick. Talk about a win-win choice!

Fructose

Don't let the word fool you. Fructose is sugar. Sometimes it's called 'fruit sugar' and, as the name implies, it comes from plant sources like tree and vine fruits, flowers, berries, and many root vegetables. Commercially, however, fructose is usually derived from sugar cane, sugar beets and maize (corn). In his book *Sweet Poison*, David Gillespie says that fructose is one of the most dangerous additions to modern processed food and one of the leading causes of obesity, diabetes and heart disease.

The main problem with fructose is our bodies have no way to determine what quantities and calories we're ingesting. When fructose is in its natural form—in an orange or an apple—it's packaged with a bunch of water and fiber. After eating an orange or two we feel full and have consumed a relatively small quantity of fructose. As you recall, fiber is the one thing that can slow down the rate at which insulin is released into the blood stream. And it's also the way the body signals the brain to "stop eating, we've had enough."

You could drink the equivalent juice of 5-10 oranges, still feel hungry, and not realize you just consumed about 20 percent of the calories you need for the day in sugar. Same thing with highly processed foods made with fructose. They can be consumed in great quantities and the body has no way to regulate the intake.

Lobbyists throw lots of money at their government representatives to stop information like this being made public. It's a big challenge finding honest information and facts about the harmful effects of sugar and fructose when there's billions of dollars to be lost if government health policy makers start recommending drastic cuts in our sugar consumption.

My recommendation
This is tough for a lot of people because they're physically addicted to these drinks. But it's one of the top things you can do to immediately improve your health:

Stop drinking ALL flavored drinks and fruit juices.

Drink non-chlorinated, unprocessed spring water and eat your fruit whole. And guess what? Limit processed foods.

The Alkaline Thing
As you have probably figured out by now, nutrition is a minefield of differing views. Even the experts can rarely agree on what is good, bad and neutral when it comes to nutrition. Hence why I've attempted to keep things as simple

as possible talking about eating philosophy and not absolutes.

What I'm about to share now is both strongly supported and strongly contested by different researchers and organizations. As always, when it comes to food, there's lots of money involved, so it's hard to determine what is fact and what is clever marketing. It's often money that speaks the loudest.

With that in mind, let's look at the principle of consuming a high alkaline diet. Medical research shows that if our blood pH varies significantly from pH 7.4, which is slightly alkaline, it can lead to illness and even death. Research also suggests diseases—including cancers—thrive in an acidic environment. Therefore, it makes sense that we want our blood to be slightly alkaline.

We can accomplish this by consuming a majority of foods and fluids which leave an alkaline by-product in the body, or alkaline ash as it is commonly referred to. At the same time we want to consume fewer foods that are acidic or leave an acidic ash. We also want to limit or reduce other activities that may increase the amount of acid in the body, like smoking, exposure to pollution, and stressful emotions.

What foods are highly alkaline?
It just so happens the foods with the highest alkalinity are among the foods with the highest nutrient content. Go figure. Maybe Mother Nature does know what She's doing. Below are some examples of some high alkaline sources:
*   Dark green leafy vegetables
*   Papaya
*   Cucumber
*   Garlic
*   Broccoli
*   Almonds
*   Olive Oil
*   Lemons, limes and grapefruit
*   Herbal teas

On the other side of the fence, highly acidic foods include:

- Artificial sweeteners
- Beef
- Pork
- Shellfish
- Alcohol
- Caffeine
- Pasta's
- Pastries
- Sugar (surprise, surprise)
- Highly processed foods (in general)

As you can see from the list of acid-forming foods, there are some big commercial food players who stand to lose a lot of money if people start reducing their consumption of beef, alcohol, caffeine and sugar. That's why I'm a little skeptical of the information available on the Internet that discounts the idea of eating a predominantly alkaline diet or a diet high in the foods that fall into the acid-forming category.

My Recommendation

I recommend a diet that consists mainly of alkaline-forming foods and, as you can see from the short list I wrote, this is in alignment with eating a nutrient-dense diet. The list of high-alkaline foods includes a lot of vegetables, nuts, fruits, and surprising things like lemons and limes. And just in case you're wondering about lemons, yes, they are slightly acidic in pH on their own. But once ingested they raise the alkalinity of the human body to 7.0 on the pH scale. Weird eh? That's why in some places lemons are called pH 'neutral.' All these foods also happen to be high in micronutrients and high in fiber.

Give rice a break

I often hear clients say they need to cut rice out of their diet because it's 'bad carbs.' These are generally clients from Western countries. The reality I have observed by living in different parts of Asia for almost 10 years now, is that a large percentage of the global population consumes rice as part of their normal diet and do fine with it. In fact, the people in these countries also have very low levels of obesity, heart disease and diabetes.

In my opinion, it's what goes with the rice that has a bigger impact on health. In Indonesia, for example, the general population consumes rice (mostly white) with almost every meal, but they also eat it **with local vegetables and minimal or no meat.** If they consume snacks, they're generally whole fruits or made from natural ingredients.

There are many different varieties of rice, like wild rice, brown rice, black, red or basmati. I always suggest eating less white rice because it's had its husk, bran and germ removed, taking important dietary fiber, vitamins and minerals along with them. White rice also breaks down faster in the body because it is processed.

Overall, there are a LOT worse choices to make than eating rice. Go for the colored rice varieties for better nutrition. I just needed to say this piece in defense of rice after hearing so many Westerners talk about how bad it is for their weight management and overall health.

What's really sad is seeing so many Indonesians adding processed foods and animal products to their diets once they become more affluent. Their health deteriorates rapidly and soon they start suffering from all the typical Western problems like heart attacks and diabetes.

This 'food' is a great condiment

I need to be careful not to stand on a soapbox with this next topic after seeing all the misinformation spread by marketing departments about it rather than information released by reputable nutritionists or research scientists. The topic?

Dairy.

My take is it's a great condiment but definitely not a health food.

From a nutritional perspective, it's high in saturated fat, sugar (lactose) and acidic in its processed form. There are also some funky studies Dr. Colin T. Campbell talks about in his book, *The China Study*, where he replicated an experiment undertaken in India.

In the experiment there were two groups of rats. One group got their protein from casein (milk protein) and the other from plant sources. Campbell then injected all the rats with a carcinogen to induce cancer. One hundred percent of the rats getting their protein from milk got cancer, and ZERO percent of rats on the plant protein diet got cancer. Now, I know that rats are different from humans. And I don't know if the study has been replicated. But that's still a pretty trippy result.

Campbell said they could turn off the cancer production in the rats on the milk protein diet when they went below five percent of their protein intake from that source.

When you think about it, how likely is it humans would normally drink HUGE quantities of milk from another animal? No other mammal on the planet drinks milk after it's weaned off mother's milk. Why us? Yes, in poverty-stricken areas, goat and sheep's milk is a welcome source of calories. But the molecular structure of goat and sheep's milk is much smaller than the molecular structure of cow milk. It's more easily assimilated by the human body and doesn't trigger the same level of allergic reactions that cow's milk does. Plus the pasteurization and homogenization of (modern) milk reduces a lot of the beneficial nutrients in the milk.

Do we really need extra calcium for strong bones using dairy as the main source like all the food ads tell us?

How do all of the herbivores, animals much bigger than us, manage the bone thing? Do they get their calcium directly from plants, nuts and seeds? You bet they do. The only other things required for good bone health are sunlight (vitamin D), exercise, and water to help maintain an alkaline pH balance and detoxify the body.

I'm cool with having the occasional cookie or cake with dairy in it. Or having some milk in a cup of tea. Or occasionally having a piece of milk chocolate (though I much prefer dark chocolate with about 85 percent cocoa). And a pizza tastes bland without a bit of cheese on top. However I don't for a minute believe I need dairy in my diet to maintain good bone health. And I certainly don't put dairy in the same category as fruit, vegetables (especially green leafy vegetables), nuts, seeds, grain, legumes, etc.

Dairy is not a health food, except for baby cows!

The Protein Myth

This is always a highly touchy subject amongst people in the health and fitness industry, and also nutritionists who come from more traditional teachings. But again, I tend to lean towards the information found in such works as Campbell's *The China Study* and supported by other medical professionals like Dr. Joel Fuhrman, Dr Dean Ornish, and Dr. Caldwell Esselstyn.

Campbell is a medical researcher who has been studying protein for over four decades. He grew up on a dairy farm, and, not surprisingly, he started out with a very strong view about the need to have significant quantities of quality animal protein in the diet. Over the years, his own laboratory studies plus extensive studies throughout the Philippines and China brought him to the conclusion that a diet high in animal protein is actually less beneficial for our health than previously thought.

Along with a number of leading researchers and physicians, Campbell suggests there is a difference between the benefits derived from animal protein and plant protein, and that plant-based protein is better for us. Plus, it has no negative side effects.

Overall, I believe the amount of protein we're lead to believe we need for optimum health is quite inflated. The multi-billion dollar protein industry, which includes meat industries, the dairy industry, and a multitude of companies producing protein bars, drinks and powders, says the amount of protein needed in the average diet is as high as 35 percent. That's a BIG difference in the numbers compared to Campbell's (and other's) less than five percent figure.

Some studies point out if a diet contains over 1500 calories per day you're automatically getting enough protein without having to go overboard with protein supplements and shakes and bars and powders and extra steaks to ensure you get enough protein to survive and thrive.

The exception for protein intake may be elite athletes, but there is some evidence that they may suffer longer-term health issues as a result of high-level consumption of protein.

Portion Sizes

When it comes to maintaining our ideal body weight and composition, one of the greatest influences, after the type of food we eat, is the amount of food we eat. The amount of calories considered necessary for normal body functioning is about 1800 calories a day for women and about 2000 for men. Depending upon lifestyles, from sedentary to highly active, and external environmental influences like climate, the calorie requirements will change.

However, one of the biggest challenges facing most people is they have no idea what an appropriate portion size is. As fast food chains have up-sized and super-sized, portions have become completely distorted. Part of the problem is that highly processed, high-calorie foods have very low fiber so we don't feel full after consuming even a large quantity. So bigger always seems better. But it's easy to blow out two-day's worth of calories with one stop at McDonald's.

When eating a diet that's more whole-food and plant-based, you have less to worry about as far as portion sizes are concerned. You're eating foods that have high fiber, natural fats and which tend to be lower in calories.

For instance, a cup of raw spinach is 7 calories, 2 tomatoes are 32 calories, 1/2 cup of cut cucumber is 8 calories, 2 tablespoons of chia seeds is 58 calories, a small handful of raw almonds is 90 calories, a tablespoon of extra virgin olive oil is 120 calories, a dash of lemon juice is 10 calories, and some organic salt and black pepper is 0 calories. We just made a nice salad at a total of 325 calories.

Compare that with one and a quarter glazed Dunkin Donuts, which also comes in at 325 calories. Which meal is likely to leave you feeling satisfied? It's a no-brainer. Plus who is likely to have the willpower to stop after eating the first quarter of a donut?

Another interesting experiment is to look at the sizes of crockery (plates, bowls and cups) from 50 years ago. A client of mine was at a local antique market and was completely amazed at how small the plates, bowls, and teacups were. As plate and cup sizes grew, so did the average size of people in Western cultures. And people 50 years ago were far more physically active! Little wonder we've got the results we have today.

Bottom line, portion sizes are generally way too big and consist of crappy 'food.' The solution is to reduce the portion sizes, especially if you're consuming meat, and increase the amount of whole plant-based food to your diet.

Salt

I eat very few processed foods so I almost forgot to include this point. However, for those who consume a higher portion of processed or fast foods, this is definitely a concern.

Excess salt (sodium chloride) can elevate blood pressure, which increases the risk of a heart attack or stroke. Plus, excess salt increases the risk of osteoporosis and even stomach cancer.

Did you know many flavored drinks and sodas are loaded with salt to make you thirstier, so you drink more? And the way they mask the taste of the excess salt is to add a bucket-load of sugar. Now that is just plain WRONG! Make no mistake; most food companies do not care about your health. So don't listen to them. See their advertisements and say, "Yeah, sure, you dodgy (beep)."

Not surprisingly, you can generally meet all your sodium needs by consuming a healthy diet of ... yes, you know what: unprocessed whole foods. So there is little need to add excess salt to your food. If you feel you must add salt, try the food first and then use only a small amount. I would also recommend you buy the most expensive high-quality organic natural salt, like Himalayan salt. There are trace minerals in it that make it better for you than processed iodized table salt. And secondly, because it is so expensive, you're likely to use it more sparingly.

You'll find as you improve your diet with natural foods, your taste buds will become more sensitive and you'll need to add fewer condiments to enjoy the flavors that are naturally occurring.

Coffee and Caffeine

Can you believe coffee is the next-most-traded commodity after oil? Makes sense because it does taste rather nice. But it's also quite a powerful stimulant, which, I think, makes it less a food source and more a drug because it artificially stimulates the body.

There's a lot of dialogue on the pros and cons of coffee for health. Dr. Joel Fuhrman, in *Super Immunity*, suggests that the positive benefits might be due to the general nutrient-poor diet of most people on a standard Western diet such that the few antioxidant properties of a coffee bean make a slight measurable positive difference. He says it might be less about the benefits of coffee and more about boosting the micronutrient quality of our diet.

For me, a cup of coffee is something to be enjoyed for the aroma, the flavor, and the company it is shared with. If you consume too much, you lose all appreciation of the flavor and may as well be drinking water (which is far better for you). The other thing is, the stimulating effects of caffeine are the result of a chemical high that makes you feel you have more energy and are more alert. But, as with any drug, the more you consume the more you need to get the same effects.

I'm all about creating energy bursts from within by moving my body, activating my mind and connecting to my breath. We have access to incredible amounts of potential power in our bodies once they're properly nourished. The better we get at accessing that power naturally, the greater the results in all areas of our lives.

Coffee is also acidic. It stains your teeth and has an internal drying effect that can exacerbate constipation.

If I were to say how much is too much coffee, I'd suggest no more than two cups (8oz or 250ml as opposed to buckets) a day. For optimum health I'd recommend drinking it occasionally as a special treat for the taste buds and a good way to connect socially. You can always opt for a glass of herbal-infused tea, which has even more additional health benefits.

One final point on coffee is the increasing amount of coffee drinks with huge amounts of added sugar and lactose from milk. For instance, a Starbucks Frappuccino is between 15-20 percent sugar—which is seriously off the charts. Drinking a black coffee, or a coffee with a dash of milk and a spoonful of sugar or honey is very different from the blended drinks, lattes, mochas, and cappuccinos when it comes to health.

A Frappé a day *does not* keep the doctor or the unwanted body fat away.

Alcohol

I can speak from very personal experience when I say that most of the worst decisions of my life were made in the company of a belly-full of alcohol. Like that time I did a back somersault off the bar at an Army Officers Ball in Sydney and almost fractured both of my heels. The pain was excruciating even with a skin-full of alcohol. I've learned I'm much wiser when I'm not drinking!

Now, on to alcohol and health. Does anyone who is not the owner of a brewery, winery, distillery or alcohol-related business believe that alcohol is essential for optimum health? Do you believe alcohol is *essential for optimum health*?

Yes, there have been some studies on the antioxidant polyphenol in red wine called resveratrol. Research with mice suggests it might help protect from obesity and diabetes and help protect the lining of blood vessels in the heart. According to the Mayo Clinic in the US, a human would have to drink about 1000 liters of red wine a day to get the equivalent doses of resveratrol used in the mice studies. Probably not a good idea.

I think we can all agree that if someone does not drink alcohol it will have no adverse health effects. Alcohol is not a nutrient, nor is it a chemical the body needs to metabolically function at its best. My recommendations on alcohol are:
1. Drink it infrequently.
2. Don't drink it in excess.
3. Drink it with plenty of water.
4. Be wary of the high-sugar mixers (coke, ginger ale, fruit juices, lemonade,

etc.). They will make you store body fat and may contribute to insulin resistance.

5. Never drink alone.
6. Stop before you lose control.
7. Get help if you have an issue with it.
8. Calculate how much you'd save in a year if you cut out alcohol, or at least cut down significantly. Consider what holiday you could have as a result. In the late 80's - early 90's, I used to spend about $10,000 a year on alcohol. And if you think that's something, add-up what three glasses of decent wine at a bar costs nowadays and multiply by 365. For the $10,000 you'll save you can have an awesome European vacation or a life-changing six-month sabbatical in Asia, even at 2014 prices!

Organic

A book on optimum health would be incomplete without a word on organic versus non-organic food. The word organic in relation to food sources means there have been no synthetic pesticides or fertilizers used, and that they're processed without the use of things like irradiation (which sounds more like a weapon of mass destruction than a food processing method), industrial solvents, food additives and dyes.

Without knowing any of the science or research, would you like to eat stuff that's been bathed in pesticides, irradiated, and mixed with solvents and other chemicals whose names you can't pronounce?

Regardless of whether there is conflicting or 'unsubstantiated' evidence to suggest that organic products have higher nutrient value, I'm definitely letting my common sense tell me organic is the better way to eat. Until science can replicate a blade of grass, I'm going to leave my trust in Mother Nature to produce the food for my body.

We'll be talking more about organic eating and living when we look at the section on detoxification.

Cholesterol

This is a fascinating subject and I am only going to highlight a few key points and then refer you to the deeply researched book written by a Ph.D. nutritionist and a cardiologist, called *The Great Cholesterol Myth*. Bowden and Sinatra's book is ESSENTIAL reading for anyone taking or considering taking cholesterol-lowering drugs. They have a huge amount of evidence to support their case that lowering cholesterol with drugs does not reduce your risk of coronary heart disease.

Obviously the 40+ billion-dollar pharmaceutical industries do not want you to know that minor point. Yes, their drugs do lower cholesterol. No, they do not reduce the incidence of coronary heart disease. And let us not forget to highlight the side effects, which include muscular pain, memory loss, and sexual dysfunction. It might be time to educate yourself and your doctor about cholesterol if you have issues with this.

Here are the basic things I took away from Bowden and Sinatra's extensive research and experience:

1. The body produces cholesterol and it is absolutely essential for the brain and body to function.
2. There is no direct correlation between lower cholesterol and lower risk of coronary heart disease.
3. Do not assume your doctor knows the full picture. Most of them are too busy to read into the subject and are too highly influenced by what the pharmaceutical industry tells them.
4. There is good cholesterol (HDL) and bad cholesterol (LDL). Bowden and Sinatra suggest that there is 'good' and 'bad' cholesterol within the LDL cholesterol. So LDL is not all bad, and a lot of cholesterol testing is not relevant.
5. They suggest the bigger danger is the excess sugar in peoples' diets coming

from ... drum roll please: highly processed foods.
6. Their recommended solution ... ratta-tat-tat: eat more whole foods.

If you have any concerns about your own cholesterol, I strongly recommend that you make a $20 investment and get yourself a copy of *The Great Cholesterol Myth* and educate yourself and your doctor. That way you can make an informed decision about your own health.

Note: I am *not* telling you to stop taking cholesterol-lowering drugs if you are on them. I am telling you to educate yourself and your doctor first and then make your own informed health choice.

Supplements

Most agricultural studies show that important nutrients found in soil are depleted by chemical pesticides, mass production, mono-cropping and over-farming. This is one of the reasons smaller organic farms are considered a much better source of nutritious foods. Again, this is up for debate by some of the bigger players in the food industry. (What a surprise.) In the meantime, knowing that most people still get their foods from factory farms, a lot of nutritionists and doctors recommend supplementation with various vitamins and mineral products.

Many nutritionists, medical professionals and homeopaths recommend a daily natural, high-quality multi-vitamin and mineral supplement as part of a healthy diet (especially for vitamin D, B12, zinc and iodine). There might also be inclusions of probiotics, digestive enzymes, magnesium, B vitamin complex, omega-3 and omega-6 supplements. But supplements are never to be used as compensation for a bad diet.

I recommend first you look at improving your diet. Once you've tightened this up and seen the impacts on your health and vitality, you might pay a visit to an integrative doctor, homeopath, naturopath or reputable nutritionist to determine if there are any gaps in your diet. But again, step one is work on the quality of your food.

Chew on this

Last, but by no means least comes the ancient art of actually chewing your food. What? No eating on the run or hovering over a meal, or standing at the kitchen counter shoveling it down? Many of us (and I am guilty of this too) see food as a fuel source that needs to get shoved in as quickly as possible so we can get on with doing something more important. But what could be more important than fueling your body and life?

When we slow down and chew our food we become more conscious of what we're putting into our bodies. We become more attuned to the flavors, aroma and texture of the food. And when it comes to our health, there are some pretty compelling reasons why we need to properly chew our food:

- Breaking down food into smaller particles aids digestion, allowing the intestines to absorb more nutrients and energy.
- Saliva contains digestive enzymes, which help break down food, making it easier for the stomach and intestines to digest and absorb.
- We tend to eat less, because taking longer to consume a meal gives the body time to relay the signals to say when we're full.
- Less energy is required for the digestion process (because of the above reasons) so we conserve energy.
- It's a healthy workout for the teeth, helping keep them strong.

By taking the time to properly chew your food you will not only get more bang for your nutritional buck, you'll also significantly reduce the likelihood of bloating, gas, wind, and other digestive problems. So, unless you are the rare human animal who already does this, I suggest you make a very conscious effort to slow down, and chew chew chew a lot more than you do.

CHAPTER 17:

Emotions and Food

When it comes to nutrition, it's important to view the body, the mind, and the emotions as a whole. Forget seeing them as separate parts. That's just more of that reductionism stuff that misses the bigger picture called you.

Our emotions affect the biochemistry of our bodies. We have a thought and that thought carries meaning and emotion. And emotion causes our brains to release different neurotransmitters, neuropeptides and hormones into our bloodstream. What we think, and therefore feel, has a physical effect on our body. Someone who worries excessively over-activates their sympathetic nervous system (stress response), potentially causing suppression of the immune system, digestive disorders, and the release of excessive amounts of cortisol into their blood steam.

If the fact that emotions affect not only the body but the food we eat surprises you, stop and think: ever had the experience of having an argument at the dinner table? It's like the food (if you can get it down) curdles right there in your stomach.

We need to not only put great food into our bodies, we need to ensure we do it in an environment as free from excessive worry and stress as possible. In line with this goal, the last thing we need is an eating regimen that itself causes us worry and stress. Not only will we not digest the foods optimally, we're less likely to extract the greatest amount of nutrient from them. Stress also creates issues with the elimination of waste from our bodies.

Which is why I teach my clients to *lean into* a healthy diet but not to get extreme or anal with it. Yes, I recommend establishing a diet that is high in nutrient-dense foods from natural sources that do not damage the environment, which are not processed, that are high in fiber and not highly acidic. And in today's world that's a big shopping list to tick off. But don't freak out and think you have to do all of it right, all the time. Everybody's lifestyle is different. It's better to eat nutrient-dense food 80 percent of the time and ease up on the other 20 percent if that helps keep you on track.

Personally, I see great benefits in a vegan raw food diet. But with my lifestyle — which includes a lot of world travel — it's just hard work trying to maintain. It requires a great deal of preparation and organization and is very restrictive. Even though eating a diet high in raw foods is undeniably great for my body, it's less stressful easing up a bit as circumstances dictate than trying to maintain this diet 100 percent of the time 24/7 and 365 days of the year.

It's important to not only to enjoy your food and get the best possible foods into your body, but you need to be able to sustain a good diet. One that's too rigid is more likely to fall by the wayside than one with a degree of flexibility. So enjoy going out with people. Enjoy trying different things. Just make the best food choices you can, each and every day. And know that being too anal, too uptight, and too preachy about the food you eat has the potential to have adverse effects on your body regardless of how great it is.

As the Buddhists teach, it's about spending most of your time in the 'middle way.' The middle path requires the least amount of energy and generates the least amount of stress. It's the way of thinking that allows the body to relax, rejuvenate and regenerate on the way to a life truly worth living.

CHAPTER 18:

The Carl Massy personal nutrition philosophy

When people ask if I'm vegetarian or vegan or some other derivative, my response is I'm not 100 percent of any label.

I was brought up on a typical Australian diet of meat and veggies, which were inevitably overcooked and great for people without teeth (sorry mum). One of the first books I read on nutrition was called *Diet for a Small Planet*, which was written by Frances Moore. (She was a vegetarian despite being told she would die from a lack of protein in her diet!) Then, in 1999, I heard Tony Robbins speak about his vegetarian diet. Given that he's 6'7" and supercharged, it opened me up to new ideas about eating.

At that point I started a vegetarian diet that included seafood. Not only did it change how I felt, it actually changed how I acted. I found myself being less aggressive and calmer. (This was also when I eased off the beers and started yoga, so it might have been a combination effect). I kept at this for about five years until I was working in Italy for the Olympic Games and it just got too hard to find non-meat cooking. So I tucked into the occasional *carne de crude* (raw mince with salt, pepper and a dash of olive oil) for something a little different.

I still ate mostly non-meat meals because I felt like I had more energy and lightness of spirit when I stuck to plant-based foods, and a big part of my diet remained fresh fruit, nuts and vegetables with minimal amounts of processed foods. When I left my security consulting life and set up my coaching business in Bali, I moved back to a whole-food plant-based diet (a term coined by Dr. Colin Campbell). Again, it just felt right for me.

But flexibility is key.

I remember on a bicycle tour around Laos I told the tour leader that I was vegetarian (an easier explanation in a foreign country). She passed the info on to the kitchen staff where we were staying. So we sit down to dinner and we're all served a whole stuffed frog! Only mine, because I was 'vegetarian,' was stuffed with a purely vegetable filling rather than a vegetable and meat filling like everyone else. What did I do? I ate it. Then I thanked my host for a wonderful meal and got on with the trip.

Today, if I'm having a meal out with my partner, who is Chinese-Indonesian, and she wants me to sample her pigeon or frog leg (not really my idea of a treat), I'll take a small portion and taste it. I know my body will be okay with this, and so I have zero stress about it. But while we're talking about meat, I'd like to take the opportunity go a little deeper into the subject.

My take on the meat thing

The choices I make on a daily basis impact the planet—from recycling my trash, to turning off light switches when I leave a room, to choosing how I travel. But one of the biggest impacts I, and the seven billion other people on the planet, have on the environment, is how and what we eat.

Currently we derive over 90 percent of our energy from fossil fuel and nuclear power, and we all know the negative effect of burning fossil fuels on the environment. Coupled with global warming, the picture gets a little grim. But here's something a lot of people don't realize. It takes at least ten times more energy to produce one serving of meat, versus one cup of grain. Not a good bang for the energy buck.

Here's another reason to reduce or eliminate meat consumption. Did you know one of the biggest pollutants on the planet is animal farts? (Also known as methane gas.) Methane is about 20 times more destructive than carbon monoxide from motor vehicles as an environmental pollutant.

And there are more environmental side effects to eating meat. Back in the day, most people couldn't afford to eat much meat. But as populations have become more affluent, the consumption of animal products and the number of livestock on the planet has exponentially increased. If not managed correctly, waste from cattle lots is a terrible pollutant of local watersheds and aquifers, passing tons of nitrates into the soil. Cows also consume vast quantities of water—which is another growing global concern.

Over three million children die of malnutrition each year. And yet there is enough food being produced, right now, to feed everyone. Yet a huge percentage of the grain, soy and corn—staple foods for large populations—are being diverted to feed livestock. And to produce these vast quantities of feed, lots of land needs to be cleared. Goodbye Amazon rainforests—the lungs of our planet converting carbon dioxide to oxygen.

Bottom line: the planet cannot sustain a global population that consumes high quantities of animal products.

Meat from an optimum health perspective

If you are an avid meat-eater and getting incensed by my dialogue on animal products, I urge you to instead be a lover of knowledge and curious about seeing a different perspective. I hope it can lead you to wisdom and more informed choices.

So, on to my recommendations about meat and optimum health:

1. A small amount of nutrients from animal-based sources is okay. I suggest less than 10 percent of your daily calorie intake from meat sources, possibly as low as five percent for optimum health and longevity. (Again, to deepen your insight, grab a copy of *The China Study*.)

2. Definitely go for organic meats as they're free from a huge range and quantity of antibiotics and hormones.

3. If possible, source your animal products locally. This means a smaller carbon footprint, more knowledge of where your food comes from, and quite possibly an even better taste.

4. Buy meats from sources that have been raised and slaughtered in an ethical way, such as grass fed or free roaming. We become what we eat.

And remember:

Don't worry so much about getting enough protein in your diet

Plant-based foods have a combination of fat, carbohydrate and protein in them. Plus they're packed with the essential micronutrients for optimum health. For example, spinach is 30 percent protein! One hundred calories of broccoli contains 11.1 grams of protein compared to 8.0 grams of protein in 100 calories worth of Porterhouse steak. Hello? If you think your bones won't grow if you don't shove a hamburger a day into your stomach, go stand beside an elephant, hippo or buffalo. If you think you won't be strong doing predominantly the plant thing, have an arm wrestle with a gorilla. Caveat: I take no responsibility for any injuries sustained while arm wrestling gorillas.

So what does my diet look like?

If you've read *The Guidebook to Happiness* you know I strongly recommend all my clients start the day with a Green Drink (also called a Green Smoothie). The base ingredient is a green leafy vegetable, like spinach or kale, adding other vegetables and fruits to flavor it (e.g. cucumber, apple, berries, banana, tomato's, prunes, chia seeds, etc.). Then you add about 600ml (20 ounces) of water (I like to use coconut water), and blend it all together. Note that it is blended and not juiced to maintain the integrity of most of the fiber.

This is a water-rich, nutrient-rich act of self-love. Seriously. From a physical and psychological level your body and mind are rejoicing as you bring this drink to your lips. I advise clients if they did nothing else in their life apart from add a daily Green Drink they would change their lives.

So, here are my general daily eating habits:

- **Breakfast.** Green Drink. About 1 liter or 33 ounces. This carries me through the morning. The ingredients are organic where possible. I also might have a few slices of papaya in the morning before I exercise.

- **Snacks.** If I'm not going to make it to lunch, I grab a small handful of raw nuts. They have the right amount of protein, fat and complex carbohydrate to keep me going and feel satisfied.

- **Lunch.** Because I live in Asia, I generally have a meal with organic rice. It is 50 percent brown rice and 50 percent white rice because my partner likes white rice. Mixed with it are some vegetables and perhaps some tempeh (a fermented soy-based product) or a tofu dish. The meal might also be a homemade miso soup, to which I add seaweed, chia seeds, flax seeds and maybe some raw nuts. Because I usually work from home, this is easy to prepare. If I'm going out for lunch, I'll either get a big plate of salad with beans and nuts, or a plate of rice and vegetables. I often eat Asian foods (Indonesian, Thai, Chinese, Japanese, and Indian) even when I'm away from Asia.

- **Afternoon snacks.** I normally have 500ml (16 ounces) of Green Drink left over from the morning. Other snacks I munch on include fruit, raw nuts, vegetables, dates, and prunes. Dried fruits aren't ideal because the water has been evaporated and they're a bit of a fructose hit. But, because they have fiber and taste great, I eat them without any guilt.

- **Dinner.** Sometimes this is a lighter meal for me. Maybe a salad with some nuts and seeds or a soup with rice. In a lot of cases it's similar to what I have for lunch.

- **Evening snack.** As I'm relaxing watching a movie, I quite often have a soda water and a piece of fruit or some dates in the evening. I might also have a couple of pieces of chocolate (I aim for over 70 percent organic dark chocolate when I go shopping).

Eating over the weekends

I'm generally more diet-relaxed on the weekends. Particularly on Sunday, which is the one-day, I don't do physical activity in the mornings. But even though I tell myself I can be more relaxed on the weekends with the food I eat, I still tend to eat pretty well.

Quite often I'll eat out on weekends—though I still start my day with a Green Drink. It's just too good to miss. I like to eat in places that have a reputation for good quality fresh and wholesome food. But overall, I just let my body (and sometimes my emotions) have a bit more say in the matter. I might have some spaghetti or a thin-crust Italian pizza with a small amount of cheese (these are very different from the thick-crusted, trans fat oil, processed, factory-farmed meat and cheese-laden pizzas you get at a Pizza Hut). Or I'll have a rice porridge, or maybe a vegetarian enchilada with less cheese, noodle soup, a salad baguette, a vegetable burger with fresh ingredients or Indonesia's signature dish, nasi goreng (fried rice).

I'm also likely to eat desserts on a weekend—a piece of good quality carrot or chocolate cake, some home-baked cookies, fried bananas, black-rice pudding or a date slice. Again, I'm cool eating this stuff. But I do prefer foods that have been made in a local kitchen as opposed to a factory hundreds (or thousands) of miles away from me and made months ago.

Fresh is best and made with love is even better!

CHAPTER 19:

Pillar 2 (Nutrition) Summary

Nutrition is one of the longest, most detailed sections in this book. These are the most important points:

1. Always aim to eat food as close to the source as possible. Straight from the garden or local green grocer to your plate would be sensational.

2. Sugar above a very low level (less than five percent of daily calories or about six teaspoons a day) becomes toxic to the body and impairs its ability to balance our metabolism. One flavored soda drink has about 8-10 teaspoons of sugar!

3. Insulin resistance is likely to result from excessive sugar intake, which can lead to the storage of excessive body fat, Type 2 Diabetes and heart disease.

4. Consuming fat is not the real demon when it comes to getting fat. The bad guy is sugar and fructose.

5. Greatly increase your intake of whole-food plant-based nutrients in your diet (fruit, vegetables, nuts, seeds, legumes and grains), because they're packed with beneficial nutrients and immune-supporting properties. These foods also contain fiber, which is essential for healthy elimination of waste, regulating blood sugar levels and fructose processing in the liver.

6. Around 80 percent of all processed foods have added sugar, artificial additives, preservatives and other chemicals, which the body cannot process and which may be toxic in larger doses. These substances may also accumulate in the body causing joint pain, swelling, inflammation and

all sorts of other problems.

7. The processing and refining of foods may also cause the body to adversely react to the modified food. I have a hypothesis that gluten intolerance is actually either created or exacerbated by the processing of grains as opposed to the grains themselves being harmful to the body.

8. Organic foods are free of pesticides, herbicides and other chemicals and treatment methods that are not supportive of optimum health. Eat organic food where possible.

9. Excessive consumption of animal products means poorer health. More work is required for the internal organs to break down and process animal products.

10. Meat products contribute heavily to the degradation of the environment.

11. Leafy greens and vegetables like broccoli are high-protein sources and regular superfoods.

12. Excessive salt consumption can lead to increased blood pressure and its knock-on effects. Most processed foods contain added salt. It's important to reduce your intake of processed foods and reduce the amount of added salt in your meals.

13. I believe dairy products are not a health food but rather a great condiment (or occasional treat). Most peoples' bodies aren't able to break down lactose efficiently or at all. The lactose in dairy products is also a sugar derived from galactose and glucose. Our bodies need less sugar, not more.

Optimum health strategies

1. Consume whole foods that are plant based. Crowd out processed foods.

2. Buy organic food where possible.

3. Stop drinking ALL flavored drinks!! Instead drink water.

4. Reduce your consumption of animal products by increasing your consumption of plant-based foods.

Recommended resources

There are many different opinions and schools of thought when it comes to nutrition. There are likely to be differences between what nutritionists and naturopaths say. In fact, there will be major differences between nutritionists depending on where they were trained and what philosophies they follow. Again, take your time finding the right nutrition counselor for you. I suggest you read some of the following books first and then seek direct support if needed.

Books:

- *The China Study* by Dr. Colin T. Campbell
- *Whole* by Dr. Colin T. Campbell
- *Eat to Live* by Dr. Joel Fuhrman
- *Super Immunity* by Dr. Joel Fuhrman
- *Dr. Dean Ornish's Program for Reversing Heart Disease* by Dr. Dean Ornish
- *Prevent and Reverse Heart Disease* by Caldwell Esselstyn
- *Sweet Poison* by David Gillespie
- *Integrative Nutrition* by Joshua Rosenthal
- *Fat Chance* by Dr. Robert Lustig
- *Why We Get Fat* by Gary Taubes
- *The Great Cholesterol Myth* by Steven Sinatra and Jonny Bowden
- *Clean Gut* by Alejandro Junger, MD
- *Finding Ultra* by Rich Roll
- *In Defense of Food* by Michael Pollan

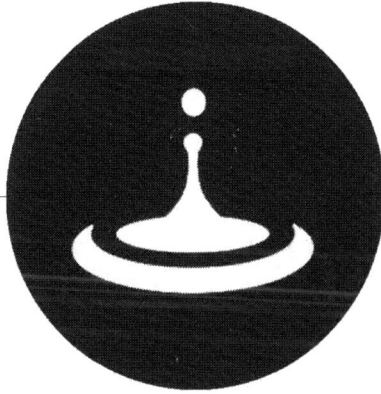

PILLAR 3
DETOXIFICATION

By cleansing your body on a regular basis and eliminating as many toxins as possible from your environment, your body can begin to heal itself, prevent disease, and become stronger and more resilient than you ever dreamed possible.
Dr. Edward Group III, alternative health specialist

CHAPTER 20:

What you don't see can still harm you

How does detoxification fit in with optimum health? Do you remember at the start of the book when I talked about creating the environment that is most conducive to the successful functioning of the body? Well, in this section we're going to be talking about how to create the best internal and external environment for the body to aid with its health.

I've studied the subject of detoxification, read books and have, as a result, introduced a number of practices into my life over the last few years aimed towards reducing both the amount of toxins my body is exposed to and the amount of toxins my body retains when it is exposed. I've experienced Ayurvedic detoxification in India and know some of the ins (and outs!) of colonics. None of this makes me an expert. For more in-depth information on detoxification I will refer you to a number of books. I also recommend you consult a naturopath or integrative medicine practitioner if you want to be supported through a formal detoxification process.

Detoxification basics

Detoxing is not reserved for someone at a rehab clinic who has abused drugs for the last 10 years. A toxin is something that causes harm to the body and synonyms for 'toxin' include poison, pollutant, and venom. I think we can all agree that for optimum health and vitality we need to reduce the amount of toxins already in our bodies and guard against those our bodies are exposed to.

The human body is naturally detoxifying all the time through our digestive, respiratory, circulatory, lymphatic and other systems. Completing some sort of detox regime is highly beneficial for us all at certain points in life.

"In Eastern traditions, one of the first things practitioners check is the ability of the body to eliminate toxins," writes Dr. Alejandro Junger in his book *Clean*. "Indian Ayurvedic doctors ... consider the ability to detoxify – to eliminate toxic waste and toxic thought and emotion – as the root source of your physical and mental health."

Toxins in the body have many sources.

First of all, they're created in the body as a result of normal metabolic functions. These are called waste products. The rest are externally introduced into our systems. In Brenda Watson's book, *The Detox Strategy*, she uses the terms *Environmental Toxins* to signify household chemicals, industrial pollutants, food additives and pesticides, and *Internal Toxins* for the by-products of normal metabolic functions. Watson also talks about things that are not normally considered toxins, but are rather foreign substances such as caffeine, alcohol and pharmaceutical drugs that the body (especially the liver) has to work extra hard to process.

If you tend to believe that most drugs aren't foreign to the body, check this out. In July 2000 the Journal of the American Medical Association (JAMA) ran an article titled "*Is US Health Really the Best in the World?*" by Dr. Barbara Starfield. In the article she cites the fact that an average 225,000 deaths occur per year in the U.S due to doctor error and the side effects of pharmaceutical drugs. That makes doctors and prescription drugs the third largest cause of deaths every year! There's even a term for it: iatrogenic (medical related) damage.

I haven't taken any pharmaceutical drugs for over a decade—no painkillers, no anti-inflammatory meds, no antacid medications or anything else. When I'm ill I take long rests, consume garlic and ginger, drink more water, remove stressors from my life, remove all processed foods and increase my intake of high alkaline plant-based foods.

The body will never perform at its optimum if it's impeded by toxins in the body or if it's constantly required to remove or neutralize toxins introduced into the body. The end result is wasted energy, an overworked and tired immune system (and other related systems in the body, such as a less efficient lymphatic system) and potential harm to the cells and organs.

Quick examples of toxins

Here are some examples of modern toxins and where they might be found. This is just a small list of the major ones to get you started:

- Asbestos – considered a carcinogen (cancer causing). This is still widely used in Asia and, I suspect, other developing countries.
- Mercury – a toxic heavy metal
- Carbon monoxide – from burning fossil fuels and lethal in large doses
- Synthetic fragrances
- Synthetic colors
- Mold

The list could go on and on. Some things may be okay in smaller doses but become toxic for the body if exposed in larger quantities.

Side effects of excessive toxicity

Here are just some of the side effects you may experience as a result of having excessive toxins in your body:

- Acne
- Allergies

- Body odor (and not the smelling like roses type)
- Fatigue
- Depression
- Digestive problems
- Insomnia
- Migraines
- High blood pressure

Ultimately, the strain put on a body's systems and organs as it attempts to process and eliminate excessive toxins can result in a massive set of symptoms and a situation that is the exact opposite of optimum health. In his book *Revive*, Dr. Frank Lipman, an integrative and functional medicine practitioner, uses the term 'spent' to describe this process of overload where people feel physically, emotionally and mentally exhausted.

The rest of the detox pillar of optimum health will educate you about:
- Ways to limit the external toxins you're exposed to.
- Ways to limit the toxins you ingest through your food and drink.
- Ways to cleanse existing toxins from the body (nobody is immune to toxicity exposure!).

CHAPTER 21:

Environmental Toxins

Reducing the amount of environmental toxins you're exposed to in our consumer society can be a pretty big job. Much of the by-product waste from manufacturing is toxic in nature. And where does it go? Into our environment in landfills that pollute ground waters and affect the soils. The plastic packaging everything, including our food, comes wrapped in is also toxic. It, too, ends up in nature—in the air we breathe, the water we drink and the soil our food is produced from.

There's only so much the world and our bodies can take.

I make a strong plea that you make an effort to reduce your consumer footprint. Owning less crap is a great way to start trimming the waste and the resultant toxins in our lives. My philosophy is that I don't have to *own* things. Whether it's a boat, a plane, a beachside villa or a tuxedo, I just lease them for the time I need them. Another solution is going in on buying things you rarely use with other people, reducing duplication. Buyers clubs save money and reduce the hassles of taking care of more stuff.

Another broad-spectrum approach to avoiding toxins is wisely choosing the place you live. Obviously you should avoid living on or near landfills, manufacturing centers, factory farms, power lines and other electromagnetic sources. Small cities and towns are generally less toxic than living in a big city. I'm currently choosing to live in Bali (Indonesia) as I like the Asian culture and professional opportunities. But I'm not about to live in one of the major cities in the region.

As far as pollution levels are concerned, countries vary. For example, Japan, with all its problems with Fukushima, is probably not the best choice right now. Unfortunately, like Chernobyl, Fukushima's radiation is spreading—not through the jet stream, but through the ocean, endangering other coastlines and nations. The more we pollute, the less easily we can escape the impact of our own shortsightedness.

Another thing to consider is the amount of toxic chemicals used in the construction of the house or apartment you live in. 'Sick Building Syndrome' is recognized as a major source of ill-health. As homes become more energy efficient and air tight, toxic chemicals off-gassing from paints and adhesives, plywood and treated lumber have more impact because they're literally sealed in with us. The cheapest way to mitigate this is to make sure your heating filters are changed regularly. And, if possible, keep some windows at least partially opened for airflow even in the winter.

Another thing to consider in the home environment is synthetic carpets, furniture and curtains off-gassing toxic chemicals. Natural fibers like cotton and wool and more neutral fibers like nylon are wise choices. As for the buildings themselves, green building products are gaining in popularity. Some homes and commercial structures in many countries are now being constructed to sustainable, green (non-toxic) standards—such as the LEED standard in the US.

The breathing thing

One of the main ways we absorb toxins is via breathing. The nasal passages are set up to capture dust particles via nasal hair (its real use as opposed to just making some people look creepy). Nasal mucus is there to trap foreign particles. Toxins in the air that are too fine to get trapped (carbon monoxide for example) go directly into the lungs where they're easily absorbed into the blood stream.

Aside from the ones already discussed, other major external environmental toxins to be aware of are ground-level ozone, carbon monoxide and particle pollution, emissions from industrial facilities and electric utilities, motor vehicle exhaust, gasoline vapors and chemical solvents. The only way to reduce our exposure to these toxins is to choose where we live, choose what we buy, choose where we work, wear appropriate safety equipment when in highly toxic environments, and be a conscious consumer.

The biggest organ in the body

Another major gateway for toxins to enter the body and get into the bloodstream is through the skin.

Did you know the skin is the largest organ in the body? Its surface area is about 21 square foot (2 square meters) and it accounts for about 15 percent of our body weight. Its principle role is to protect the body from pathogens and water loss. It also helps regulate body temperature, synthesizes vitamin D and insulates the body.

Whether chemicals or toxins pass through the protective layer of skin is dependent on the molecule size and the solubility of the chemical, the condition of the skin and the thickness of the skin, which is much thicker on our hands and feet than it is under our arms or on our eyelids.

Not everything that touches our skin penetrates. But we do want to remain conscious of what we use. From hair care products, to deodorants, to soaps, to laundry detergents and household chemicals, a lot of products are safe and a lot of products aren't safe. Remember, just because something's on the shelf in the supermarket doesn't mean it's good for you.

Check online for comprehensive lists of chemicals in skincare and cosmetic products to avoid. There are a ton of health sites talking about this.

Carl Massy's beauty tips

Yes, I know, I'm hardly the person to be giving beauty tips. But just humor me and I'll reveal what I've experienced over the last decade when it comes to cosmetic and personal hygiene products. Yes, it's coming from the perspective of a dude. But at least it's from personal experience.

You may be alarmed to hear this, but I haven't used an underarm deodorant for about 15 years. Here's why. First, the skin under our arms is very thin, sensitive and way too close to a major lymph node under each arm. So I'm not big on chemical experiments taking place there — like adding aluminum from an antiperspirant. Imagine clogging your pores with something that's great for making boats so you don't smell. Does that sound weird to you as well?

Rather than clogging my pores with aluminum or masking my odors with a fragrance, I *address the root cause of body odor.*

When I eat a healthy whole-food plant-based diet, drink plenty of water and exercise; I don't stink. No one does if they've detoxed their body and are conscious of their diet. The times I do have a less-than-pleasant fragrance is if I consume alcohol, eat processed or junk food, eat a lot of meat and animal products, don't shower regularly and wear my shirts numerous days in a row.

This is what I mean about making lifestyle changes. And just in case you're having second thoughts about that deodorant spray you just bought, think about the toxic propellants it releases into the atmosphere with each spray. Consider Brenda Watson's point in her book *The Detox Strategy*: "Because parabens are used in commercial deodorants, particularly antiperspirants, scientists are now considering a link between the use of common deodorants and an increased risk of breast cancer in women."

Remember, once upon a time fragrances and cosmetics were made from natural ingredients. I'm quite certain the Egyptians, Persians, Romans and Arabs did not create their most lavish fragrances in a chemical laboratory. Now there's a whole natural cosmetic industry digging up roots and picking leaves to put in everything from shampoo to toothpaste. Speaking of which, ditch the toothpaste with fluoride. It's been linked to everything from cardiovascular disease to cancer.

Household products

Yes, there are criteria to meet before a cleaning product can come to market. But a lot of times the studies are conducted over a limited time period measured in months or a few years rather than looking at decades and a lifetime of use and build-up. Another challenge in this modern age is the sheer amount of synthetic chemicals and toxins we're exposed to. Maybe one product is okay for your skin (as verified via stringent research and testing). However, when used at the same time as five other synthetic products, the effect might be very different than the laboratory results!

I deal with this situation by always choosing cleansers made from natural ingredients. I also make choices that limit my exposure to different chemicals. For instance, instead of slathering my body with a commercial sunscreen I wear a hat, protective clothes, and stay in the sun for shorter periods of time. When it comes to laundry detergents, again, I use a natural product. My clothes will be up against my skin all day unless I work nude. (Just joking!) So it's important they don't contain chemicals.

A number of years ago I was talking to my auntie Lyn (who is not a hippie, a greenie, or New Age woman, but just a normal intelligent house-owner). She told me she'd removed all household chemicals and cleaning products. In their place she used the three best natural ingredients for household cleaning — white vinegar, baking soda and lemon juice — which are just as effective as any commercial product and not toxic for your body or your loved ones'.

Just mix equal parts of vinegar and water in a squirt bottle and use it to clean kitchen and bathroom surfaces. It also disinfects and deodorizes. And don't worry; the smell disappears when the solution dries. Just make sure you do a little trial with the liquid before you put it onto specialty surfaces like marble.

There are numerous sites on the Internet that give you very clear and practical advice on how to remove household chemicals and replace them with natural ingredients. Again, this is about lifestyle choices and changes. You don't have to do all this overnight. But the sooner you stop contaminating your body the better.

Do a little research. Find out what works for you. Simplify your life. You'll not only consume less but you'll help create less market need for superfluous stuff. Plus, you'll find you need less income to maintain your lifestyle. The knock-on effect can mean you can work fewer hours, have more rest, get to spend more time with friends and family, have less stress and therefore optimize your health.

Sounds like a good plan to me.

CHAPTER 22:

Food and Drink

Some information in this section might seem a bit of a repetition on points we discussed in nutrition. But that's how we learn so I'll stick with it and hope you do too.

It will come as no surprise that a major key to minimizing the toxins that end up in your body is to eat organic whole foods where possible. Today, the largest growth rate of any agricultural sector is the organic market. Farmers can't keep up with the demand because there aren't enough organic farmers. And the reason there aren't enough organic farmers is because it takes an average of seven to ten years to switch a farm using synthetic fertilizers and chemicals to commercial organic status, and most farmer's can't afford to stay out of commercial production that long.

That's right, it takes about a *decade* to get that crap out of the soil. Is it any wonder it takes time to detox our bodies?

Of course, other things at the top of the 'not good for you' food list are artificial sweeteners (e.g. aspartame), artificial colors, preservatives, trans fat (an artificially created fat – e.g. partially hydrogenated vegetable oil), and additives like MSG. The only thing these 'foods' have in common is that none of them exist in nature—not in fruits, vegetables, nuts, seeds or legumes. They're all man-made toxic elements that exist in processed foods.

I also avoid genetically modified (GM) foods. The Artic Apple has been genetically modified to not brown after its cut. It might still *look* healthy three weeks later in the fridge. But is it really good to eat? And why do I care if it browns? Isn't the whole point of an apple to just eat it?

There's a lot of information flying around on the Internet and in print about the pro's and cons of GM foods. It's a very big business and at times quite unethical. I'm a bit of a purist, I admit. But I lived for two years in Greece which is legally GM free, and the produce there was awesome.

Trying to grow bigger crops through GM intervention is treating the symptom, not the cause. If we want to remove world hunger, we need to review the eating habits in developed and developing countries. The perceived shortage of food globally is more about the redirection of crops to feed livestock for the more affluent than anything else. And the amount of food wastage in developed countries is significant. The U.S. throws out $165 billion worth of food every year — 40 percent of what's sold in stores and restaurants.

Meat

From a toxicity standpoint, one of the biggest downsides to consuming meat is the chemicals in the feed ingested by factory-farmed animals. That and the antibiotics they're shot with because their living conditions are so crowded and unsanitary. Even their feed grains are laced with antibiotics. The difference between organic grass-fed free-range beef and mass-produced beef is huge. The same goes for mass-produced poultry, pork, lamb, etc.

Which brings me around to the most overused, deceptive word in modern food marketing today: natural.

Don't let the words 'natural' and 'all natural' on packaging fool you. Cyanide is 'natural.' But that doesn't mean you want to eat it. 'Natural meats' usually means livestock are not raised using antibiotics. But their feed is still not organic.

'All Natural' is prominently displayed on the packaging of thousands of items in the processed food sections and many of these products contain dozens of chemicals—sodium diacetate and potassium bromate and aluminum phosphate and calcium phosphate monobasic, just to name a few. Just because aluminum and phosphates are mined right here on good ol' planet Earth doesn't mean they belong in our stomachs.

Which brings up another huge subject: cookware.

Do NOT use aluminum cookware. Do not use Teflon and other synthetic non-stick pots and pans or utensils. Use stainless steel or ceramic-coated kitchenware.

Bottom line, by increasing the amount of whole organic vegetables, fruits, nuts, grains, seeds, and legumes in your diet, reducing your animal product consumption (and making what you do eat organic), eliminating highly processed foods and using high quality pots and pans you will definitely be getting less toxins into your body while boosting your immune system.

Fish and Seafood

The topic of fish and seafood is a pretty big, especially when you bring in the over-farming of our oceans. My general take on fish and seafood is the following:

1. As waterways (inland and the ocean) become more polluted, all fish and seafood are likely to carry different toxins in their bodies (like mercury and other heavy metals).

2. Farmed fish are not all that healthy. They live in over-populated tanks, swimming in their own poop, are fed questionable foods and often live in chlorinated, fluoride-laden waters. Farmed salmon is frequently injected with artificial coloring to make the meat appear normal. So get to know where your fish is coming from.

3. Smaller fish like sardines are likely to have ingested less heavy metals and may be a better choice than larger fish like tuna.

The last word on beverages

The first word is **skip all flovoured drinks** and soda's on the market. If they don't have any *chemical* toxins, they all have processed sugar or sugar's evil cousins, artificially extracted fructose and artificial sweeteners, in them. So choose water as your primary drink.

When it comes to water, again, some choices are better than others.

If you're not living on a private well, it's a good investment to get a good quality water filter. The problem with buying bottled water is the inordinate amount of plastic wastage (plus the environmental pollution of producing the plastic bottles). Also there is tremendous evidence on the negative health impacts of BPA and other plastics on the human body that leach from these bottles. So definitely invest in a good quality filter for city tap water in preference to drinking bottled filtered or spring water.

If you are living on a private well, be sure to get your water tested every couple of years because of increasing groundwater pollution.

CHAPTER 23:

Detoxification the simple way

Even though we know some things are great for us a lot of times we just don't do them. One of the most common reasons (excuses!) is, "Yes, I know this is good for me *but*, I don't have time."

Well, it's going to be hard to use that excuse when I tell you one of the most simple detox strategies you can use takes less than 0.7 percent of your day to complete. Do you have less than one percent of your day to commit to a lifestyle practice that increases your energy, improves your health, helps cleanse your body, helps with waste elimination, hydrates your body and makes you feel good about yourself?

If I'm getting any no's at this stage, we really have to discuss what else you're packing into your day. And I need to know what tricks you have up your sleeve that have a higher health return on investment (HROI) than what I'm offering you. So, are you ready for my magical detox strategy?

Enter, stage left, the humble *Green Drink* I mentioned earlier. Drinking a daily Green Drink is one of the top detox strategies I teach all of my clients in all my seminars. It's a high-fiber, micronutrient, water-rich, alkaline, life-giving, wonder drink that packs a punch like you wouldn't believe.

A typical Green Drink might include:

- Base ingredients: Dark green leafy vegetables like kale, collards, spinach and Bok Choy.
- Sweetener: Add fruit as you like — apple, banana, berries, papaya, melons, etc.
- Water (or fresh coconut water if you have access to it, since it is an awesome electrolyte drink).
- Any other superfoods you want to add, such as spirulina, maca powder, acai juice or berries, chia seeds, cacao, goji berries, hemp seeds, aloe vera, chlorella, and wheatgrass.

Elimination of waste is a HUGE part of the detoxification process, so the Green Drink is made in a blender, not a juicer, which means it retains most of the fiber from the ingredients essential for elimination of waste via the bowels. The other thing that helps with elimination is water added to the drink. If we become dehydrated, our body pulls water from the bowels, affecting our ability to poop and remove wastes. If you're someone who has any constipation issues then a daily Green Drink will definitely help.

The dark green leafy vegetables used as the base ingredient in the Green Drink are very high in nutrient value but low in calories. Dr. Joel Fuhrman, (*Super Immunity*), considers kale to be the number one nutrient-dense food because of the amount of micronutrients it has versus the calories per gram. Kale has a huge ROI. The fruits chosen to sweeten the Green Drink are also high in nutrient value and antioxidants. Plus, they are water-rich, which is again aiding with hydration and elimination. Any other superfoods you add to the Green Drink increases the nutrient and antioxidant density of the drink, so you get even more benefit.

For many thousands of years Indian Yogi's have said that when we eat food we take in the prana (or energy) of that food. We're not just talking calories, but the actual 'life-force' of the food. Not surprisingly, prana is deemed strongest in live foods such as freshly picked fruits and vegetables, as opposed to 'dead' foods like processed meals or meat. They suggest that whatever you ingest you inherent the energy (or deadness and lack of energy) accordingly.

From a science perspective there is some conjecture over the validity of these claims. But from a personal and practical level I can say there is definitely something at work when you eat live foods versus dead foods. In workshops I get people to slowly and consciously eat a piece of apple. Then I have them slowly and consciously eat a piece of chocolate. Most people agree both have great flavors, but that the apple seems to have more layers and depth to it. There is more going on when eating the apple than just a flavor sensation.

The word 'vitality' seems to describe this sensation of something 'more.' When I drink a Green Drink I feel more vital. I feel more energetic at a subtle level. I immediately have a buzz going on. Perhaps it's the macronutrients, micronutrients or the additional fluid coming into my body. Or perhaps it's something more, especially since the effect is instantaneous. Regardless of whether you believe the scientists or the yogis, try it for yourself and let your body be the judge.

Even more feel good

The other great detox benefit of a Green Drink is psychological. Taking the time to prepare and drink something that you know is great for your body is an act of self-love that goes a long way towards counteracting the many negative thoughts we all have about ourselves every day.

And have no doubt; your body can sense the goodness of food before it even enters your mouth.

Dr. David Hawkins, psychiatrist and author of *Power vs. Force*, talks about an experiment he performed in his seminars revealing the human body's capacity to intelligently 'read' the energy information of substances before they're introduced into the body. In the experiment he handed sealed envelopes containing either an artificial sweetener or a natural sweetener to attendees.

He then used kinesiology, also known as 'muscle testing,' on the person while s/he held the envelope against their body. Students' muscles would go weak when they held the envelop of artificial sweetener and their muscles would test strong when a natural sweetener was in the envelope. The body (the brain and nervous system) just 'knew' which sweetener was artificial and harmful and which was natural and healthy and responded accordingly.

I think the same thing happens when we bring the Green Drink to our lips. Our bodies' cells are already celebrating. They know a dose of pure goodness is about to come inside. Talk about a self-love hit! It's one of the key things I work on when coaching my clients. The more we love ourselves, the better we take care of ourselves on every level.

Green Drink Recipe

Equipment: Blender. You can either go for a top-of-the-range blender or a $50 job. Get what works and fits your budget.

1. Good handful of kale, spinach, collards or other dark green leafy vegetable (you might have to play around to get the best type or combination).
2. One apple
3. 1/3 cucumber
4. 1 tomato (optional—I like tomato. Remember, it's a fruit.)
5. 1 banana (peel and then freeze to add coolness to the drink)
6. 1 cup of papaya
7. 20 ounces (600ml / 1 pint) of water or fresh coconut water

Put the greens in the blender followed by all of the roughly chopped fruit and finally the water or coconut water. Blend into a smooth consistency. Drink immediately. I also save a portion of my Green Drink for later in the afternoon in case I hit a slump. Consume the Green Drink within 12 hours. If you keep it longer than this it may go off and/or lose energetic potency.

A great way to speed up preparation is to chop the fruit the night before. You can keep a container of chopped fruit in the fridge for 3-4 days worth of Green Drinks. I also recommend drinking the Green Drink first thing in the morning to set you up for the day ahead.

Because the food is processed by the blender, it allows the digestive system time to have an extended rest (well over 12 hours) from dinner time until midday when I eat a solid meal again. Less energy required for digestion equals more energy available for me to live my life and for my body to put towards repair and recovery.

CHAPTER 24:

Doing the Detox Thing

Here are a number of additional suggestions on how to detoxify your body in order to experience a higher level of health and vitality.

Detoxify your environment

If you're living in a big city it's a good idea to buy an air purifier. You can also use household plants to aid with cleaning the air. Brenda Watson, author of *The Ultimate Health Secret*, suggests spider plants, aloe vera, chrysanthemum, Gerber daisies, fern, ivy and philodendrons. (I hope these plant names mean more to you than me!)

As quickly as you can, reduce, or remove, all household chemicals and replace them with natural alternatives like vinegar, baking soda and lemon juice. You might start with the kitchen, then the bathroom, and finally the rest of the house. Don't forget to address the laundry detergent you use.

We've talked about using natural soaps and cosmetics. You can also search online for how to make natural products, including toothpaste. A simple one is just mix baking soda with coconut oil. The baking soda neutralizes the acid build up around the teeth, flossing and brushing removes the physical residue of plaque, and the coconut oil kills bacteria. You can also add a couple drops of a natural peppermint oil to get that minty taste in your mouth happening.

There are other simple things you can do to improve the health of your home environment, such as letting in as much natural light as possible. This helps with the body's natural circadian rhythms and puts you more in touch with nature.

Switch from plastic to glass storage containers, especially to store hot or heated food. Personally I'm not a fan of microwave ovens. I have a very intelligent friend who explained, at great length, the scientific process that's occurring when food is microwaved in order to show me how safe it is. However, when I asked if he'd go so far as to recommend mothers heating up their breast milk in a microwave and feeding it to their babies, he balked. (One reason is that microwaves heat unevenly and some babies have been scalded drinking microwaved milk that had 'hot spots.')

Yes, there is a lot of scientific information touting the safety of microwaves. And there are also studies showing that it changes the chemical structure of the food you eat. For sure, microwave ovens are responsible for many carcinogenic toxins leaching out of plastic packaging and containers into your food. Packaged microwavable pizzas, popcorn and 'heat 'n eat' dishes release polyethylene terephthalate (PET), benzene, toluene, and xylene. Microwaving fatty foods in plastic containers leads to the release of dioxins.

Not what you're looking for on the path to optimal health!

Detoxifying with food

You now know the basics of what to eat and what not to eat. But it helps to know that some foods are more affected by herbicides and pesticides than others. For instance, a banana is less likely to contain pesticides in its flesh than a strawberry, which has a very thin and permeable skin. Therefore, some foods you really need to buy organic. For a list of fruits and vegetables that are most likely to contain excessive toxins, check out the Environmental Working Group's website (www.ewg.org) where they list *The Dirty Dozen Plus*.

The original Dirty Dozen includes (in 2013):

- Apples
- Strawberries
- Grapes
- Celery
- Peaches
- Spinach
- Sweet Bell Peppers
- Nectarines
- Cucumbers
- Cherry Tomatoes
- Snap Peas
- Potatoes
- Hot Peppers
- Kale

Detoxifying Foods

There are a number of foods that actually contribute to the detoxification of your body while you maintain a normal eating regime. These foods are effective because they provide antioxidants, soluble and insoluble fiber, vitamins, minerals, monounsaturated fat, anti-inflammatories, phytonutrients, chlorophyll, enzymes, essential amino acids, and omega-3 fatty acid. A list of the common detoxifying foods (which are generally the nutritional superfoods) are:

- Pomegranate
- Garlic
- Seaweeds
- Lemons
- Apples
- Cabbage
- Quinoa
- Wheatgrass

- Almonds
- Avocados
- Blueberries
- Ginger
- Beets
- Green Tea
- Flaxseeds
- Dandelions
- Broccoli
- Kale
- Grapefruit
- Lemongrass

Foods to eliminate

If you're serious about cleansing your body you need to cut certain things out of your diet during a cleanse period. This includes: caffeine, alcohol, sugar, processed foods, fried foods, dairy and animal products. Gluten can also be a problem substance for a number of people and is mainly in wheat and other processed grain products.

Probiotics

Probiotics are live microorganisms (mostly bacteria) and are similar to the good microorganisms naturally found in the stomach and digestive organs. They are essential to healthy digestion and the processing of our food. These good bacteria are great for supporting the immune system and preventing conditions that negatively affect the gastrointestinal tract. *The Institute for Integrative Nutrition* suggests that eating whole foods that naturally contain probiotics is key to good health.

Probiotic rich foods include yogurt, kefir, lacto-fermented sauerkraut, miso, tempeh, kombucha, kimchi, pickles, and microalgae like spirulina, chlorella, and blue-green algae. Just make sure you read the labels when purchasing these food items to confirm that they contain *active live cultures*. A lot of yogurts are heat-treated or pasteurized resulting in the loss of the active live cultures, plus most of them are loaded with sugar and stripped of healthy fats. So be selective with yogurt. And don't consume a tub at a time or it stops being as beneficial.

For more information on the role that probiotics play in our health, check out the book *Integrative Nutrition* by Joshua Rosenthal.

Drink the good stuff

Want to detoxify your body each and every day? Cut down or eliminate caffeine. Caffeine drinks are diuretics, which means they increase the excretion of water from the body—not what we're after when it comes to detoxing and cleansing. More than two regular cups (250ml or 8 ounces) a day is when things start to become less than beneficial.

Drink more water. This will help your body flush out toxins and also keep your bowel movements more regular, which is essential for optimum health. And remember, the more caffeine you drink the more water you need to consume to balance out its drying effects.

Supplements

To support the detox process you might include a daily multi-vitamin and mineral supplement, plus a mix of different natural supplements to aid in purification and elimination such as probiotics, digestive enzymes, herbs called adaptogens, and additional vitamins and minerals.

It's a good idea to consult a naturopath, homeopath or a detox specialist to get a specific idea of the supplements that will support a detox process as it specifically relates to you.

Pharmaceutical drugs

One of the problems of detoxing while on pharmaceutical drugs is that apart from numerous potential side effects they interfere with the internal flora (bacteria) in the stomach, killing a lot of good bacteria and creating an imbalance of flora in your stomach. This has numerous knock-on effects.

One of the worst offenders is antibiotics, which, I think, are generally overprescribed. They play havoc on the internal flora and it may take months and years to get the flora back to normal if you don't formally address it. If you've had a cycle of antibiotics I definitely recommend doing a formal detox. Eating probiotic foods is also a must.

IMPORTANT: I'm not saying you should go off your meds. If you're currently on prescription medication you must do your best to compensate. But you may also be surprised if you take the detox thing seriously and really go at it that your need for medication for many different ailments will be decreased tremendously, if not potentially eliminated.

Physical Activity

Physical activity is essential to the detoxification of the body by assisting the operation of the lymphatic system through contraction of muscles massaging the internal organs to increase blood flow, thus maintaining a healthy cardiovascular system and reducing the amount of fatty tissue which can be a storehouse for different toxins

Rest

The body needs to rest in order to do repair and maintenance work at a cellular and system level. So getting a good nights rest (7.5 – 9 hours) is essential for the body to do its work. Plus, resting throughout the day with mini-breaks will aid the body's ability to detox.

Mindfulness

There is a direct relationship between toxic thinking and the toxicity of our bodies. It's very hard to separate our thinking from the physical function of the body. Our thinking and emotions have a huge impact, triggering the release of neurotransmitters, neuropeptides and hormones into the blood stream. Negative thinking and the biochemical responses initiated by it create more acid in our bodies. If our thoughts are positive, flowing, compassionate and loving we're going to experience a healing biochemical cocktail that cleanses the body.

By practicing mindfulness techniques we can deactivate the stress response and engage the relaxation response which supports repair, rejuvenation and maintenance work within our bodies. So meditation and breathing exercises are definitely related to detoxing.

Massages

I'm a huge fan of massages. They're not only great for relaxing and de-stressing, but also great for increasing blood flow through our muscles and internal organs. This increased blood flow aids in the detoxification process. Plus they feel great! It's hard to overthink and stress-out when you are blissing-out on the massage table.

Formal Detoxification Programs

Hopefully, by now the benefits of detoxifying are clear to you. I'm not a detox expert or specialist, which is why I've given you an overview and not included a specific plan for a major detox program. There is a list of online resources and books to point you in the right direction at the end of this section.

I highly recommend taking the time out each year to do a cleanse for the body. Whether you do an at-home, self-managed detoxification program, join a detox retreat or go to a specialist detoxification center for a complete overhaul, the most important thing is doing it.

The ideal detoxification process will not only focus on the physical, but also deal with the mental and emotional components for a full lifestyle audit. As you will see in the following pillars on mindfulness and wholeheartedness, working solely on the body and neglecting the mind and heart (emotions) will not be anywhere near as effective as a program that addresses all three.

One final note: detoxing doesn't have to mean a boring week spent with your juicer and the toilet. One of the greatest detoxes I've done in recent years was a one-week trek in Nepal. Once we got into the mountains, we ate only vegetarian food which was picked from gardens out back of most restaurants. We breathed fresh mountain air and kept physical throughout the day. We were free of technology and, because there were no televisions in the lodges where we stayed each night, we tended to converse more and retire early. No worries, no stress. Just life at its best.

If you want a great kick-start to initiate a healthy lifestyle, I highly recommend a vacation like this one. The company we used, which was awesome, was *Hemingway's Journeys*.

CHAPTER 25:

Detoxing and Weight Loss

I bet you didn't know that it's a lot harder to lose weight if your body is filled with toxins. In fact, your body will actually *retain* weight.

Have I got your attention now?

I know I do! So, why is this the case? Well, it's a combination of factors. One of the ways the body removes toxins from the blood is to store them in fat cells. Great move by the body, not so great for weight loss. The body is wired to not release the fat cells because by doing so it would release a lot of toxins into the bloodstream and make you very sick. So the body retains the fat cells.

Maybe you're thinking, "that's okay, I'll just train harder in the gym to burn off those fat cells by pressing the 'fat-burning' program on the step machine." Good in theory, but do you know what one of the by-products of exercise is? Lactic acid. Theoretically you produce less lactic acid if you're doing a fat-burning (low heart rate) based activity. But you're still creating lactic acid.

Remember about the alkaline and acid levels of the blood and how we need our blood pH to be slightly alkaline? *If our pH goes too far either way we can die.* Due to external pollution, stress and the acid foods we eat, most peoples' whole system is already far too acidic for good health to occur. The last thing your body wants to do is add a load of toxins and more acids to your system by burning off those fat cells.

For those of you who smash yourselves at the gym for two hours every day trying to lose weight and yet find it never really shifts, now you know what might be happening. The body can't release the fat cells because that would spike the acid levels in your blood. So exercising harder is definitely not the way out.

Before you throw your arms up in the air in despair, let me share what I believe to be a great strategy for long-term weight loss and weight management.

1. Commit to a long-term plan. This means coming into the weight loss thing with the knowledge that there MUST BE A LIFESTYLE (and mindset) change.

2. Start making lifestyle changes based on the information in this Guidebook. Start making small changes and build up from there. Don't overdo it at the start or you'll be overwhelmed and tend to slide back into your old lifestyle habits for comfort. Remember, you're committing to optimum health for the rest of your life.

3. Start detoxing body and mind. We'll get more into the mind later in the book. But know that the body and mind are invariably linked to a degree science is only now beginning to comprehend.

4. Start with a more intense detoxification, like a formal 6-8 day detox retreat or the like if you can. Or follow one of the cleanses outlined in books on detoxing (*Cleanse* by Dr. Alejandro Junger is a great example). You're likely to shed a number of pounds through this process.

5. Increase the amount of alkaline-based foods you're getting into your diet. Whole-foods and plant-based foods are a good place to start. Make sure you're consuming plenty of water and step up the amount you drink during the cleanse process.

6. A daily Green Drink is a must at this point.

7. Get in the habit of showing up for some physical activity most days of the week. Depending on where you're starting, that may be as little as going for a ten-minute walk or doing a 45-minute powerwalk.

8. Bring more consciousness into your life by being aware of what you eat, aware of what you do, aware of what you think, aware of your habits, aware of your emotions and how you process them - or how you stuff them away. The more consciousness you bring to your life the better decisions you'll make in every moment.

CHAPTER 26:

Pillar 3 (Detoxification) Summary

When it comes to Detoxification, these are the most important points for Optimal Health

1. Eat organic produce whenever you can to reduce the amount of toxins you are ingesting.

2. Buy locally produced foods to reduce the amount of energy required delivering it to your table.

3. Cut out or significantly reduce your intake of processed foods (less than 10 percent of all food).

4. Chemicals are absorbed through the skin, so aim to reduce the amount of chemicals you put on your body and buy natural products.

5. Reduce the amount of toxins in your household by removing toxic cleaning products and using more natural sources like lemon, vinegar and baking soda.

6. Do a mini daily detox (and get a mega dose of micronutrients into your body) by having a daily Green Drink. This will provide the body significant rest time between the last solid meal of the previous day and the first solid meal of the new day, which will aide with cleansing your system. Check out www.theguidebookseries.com for a simple recipe.

7. Pollutants, toxins and the use of pharmaceutical drugs negatively impact our internal gut flora. Ways to improve the internal flora include removing processed foods, sugar, gluten and dairy from your diet plus increasing the amount of probiotic and enzyme-rich food.

8. Flavored beverages are TERRIBLE for your health. They're packed with toxic sugar or fructose and other additives, preservatives and unhealthy chemicals. Remove them from your diet.

9. Do a formal detox once a year. It's incredibly beneficial to your health. Investigate a detox program either from the resources I have listed or get online and check out a good quality detox retreat.

10. When you buy stuff you don't really need, you're adding to the pollution of the planet, so purchase consciously. You'll feel better and so will the planet.

Optimum Health Strategies

1. Have a daily Green Drink.
2. Buy organic, local, and in-season produce.
3. Don't buy crap you don't need. Spend your money consciously.
4. Progressively reduce, with an aim to eliminate, toxic chemicals in your household, bathroom and make-up draw (that one is mainly for the ladies). Use or buy natural products.
5. Investigate a detox program either from the resources I have listed or get online and check out a good quality detox retreat.

Recommended Resources

Tyler Tolman is a pioneer in detoxing both body and mind. He runs intensive detox programs in Bali and supported programs online.
www.tylertolman.com

Books:

- *Clean – Expanded Edition* by Dr. Alejandro Junger
- *Clean Gut* by Dr. Alejandro Junger
- *The Detox Strategy* by Brenda Watson, C.N.C.
- *Integrative Nutrition* by Joshua Rosenthal

Websites:

- www.globalhealingcenter.com (with Dr Group)
- www.bembu.com
- www.tylertolman.com (with Tyler Tolman)

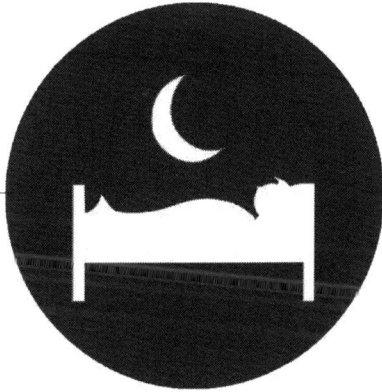

PILLAR 4
REST

Sleep is that golden chain that ties health and our bodies together.
Thomas Dekker, English dramatist

CHAPTER 27:

Rest up or fall down

This was actually the first chapter I started writing. The subject is relatively straightforward, I'd just interviewed a sleep coach and had gotten the recommended 7.5 hours sleep the night before. Plus, it's a favorite subject of mine. What better time and place to kick my writing habits into gear?

RANDOM TIP: Beginning with something fun or something you know you have a high probability of completing successfully is a great strategy for creating momentum for any project start, big or small. When we succeed at something we get a good feeling compliments of some brain chemicals like dopamine. The body gets attached to that chemical feeling and the process that triggered it. As you know, we're highly influenced by pleasure and pain, so why not use it?

Now, back to the subject at hand.

Rest seems such a simple subject. We need it. It normally happens at night. If we don't get enough then we feel like crap. But I want to deepen your understanding of how critical rest is and how completely it's tied into optimum health.

A high percentage of people in all the developed countries are sleep deprived. Over 30 percent of adults and 31 percent of teens in the U.S. get significantly less sleep than recommended. According to the NIH (National Institutes of Health) up to 15 percent of all adults suffer from chronic insomnia and up to

40 percent experience insomnia symptoms during the course of any given year. These statistics are likely to be typical in most other western and developing countries.

Personally, I believe a lot of this is due to the incredible number of distractions we experience nowadays. Our attention is pulled in thousands of different directions by phones, text messages, advertising, media, TVs and the fast pace of modern life. In this over-stimulated environment we need to get MORE rest on a daily, weekly, monthly and yearly basis. And yet the trend is towards getting less and less.

Sleep basics

Sleep is super important for optimum functioning of the body. Sleep gives the heart a well-earned break by lowering the resting heart rate. It relaxes the muscles of the body to allow for repair and replacement of cells with their trillions of functions. It allows the major organs to perform the cleansing and clearing of waste and toxins from the body in preparation for elimination.

There are two main types of sleep and they occur in a cyclical pattern lasting about 90 minutes each about 4-6 times each night (depending on how long you sleep):

1. **Non-REM** sleep (3 stages): transition to sleep (first 5 minutes), light sleep (next 10 – 25 minutes), and deep sleep.

2. **REM** (rapid eye movement) sleep: when you have your most interesting (and if you're lucky) dreams where you're a superstar, loved by the masses and have a great girl (or guy) fall into your arms. REM sleep happens about 70-90 minutes after you fall asleep.

In simplistic terms, non-REM deep sleep rejuvenates the body and REM Sleep rejuvenates the mind. So it's vital for the body and mind to have enough time to cycle through adequate deep sleep and REM sleep.

Eighty percent of adults need 7.5 to nine hours sleep per day. Less than about seven hours adversely affects most people, triggering loss of concentration, creativity, physical vitality, and mental sharpness.

In a lot of ways the mind is like a muscle. It needs fuel and it needs downtime so it can process the billions of sensory inputs you had during the day. During REM sleep the brain decides what information to take from short-term memory and convert to longer-term memory. 'Brain fog' or being 'out of it' are essentially the end result of not allowing the brain adequate opportunity to do its sorting, storing and discarding.

When we get enough REM sleep our mind is not cluttered with useless information. We're able to be more creative. Our problem solving abilities are enhanced. We're less reactive. We can more easily focus on the things we want—like picturing thoughts that enhance our mood and wellbeing and being able to form a clear mental picture of the goals and desires we have for the day ahead.

Sometimes when we're getting foggy it helps to just close the eyes and reduce the sensory input and decoding work associated with vision, thus freeing up a large portion of the brain to do its work.

Dancing with Serotonin and Melatonin

I'm forever amazed at the beautiful symphony that occurs inside our bodies. It's absolutely miraculous and I sincerely hope by the end of this book you'll have developed a similar appreciation. The amount of incredible functions taking place while we lie back on the couch with our feet up, or comfortably sleeping at night, is nothing short of miraculous. Which brings me around to two key players in the whole rest thing: melatonin and serotonin.

Often the *quality* of our sleep has a bigger impact on our waking hours than the total number of hours sleep we get. And much of the quality of our sleep is determined by how effectively our brains produce these two essential chemicals.

Melatonin is the main hormone produced from the neurotransmitter serotonin and secreted by the pineal gland near the center of the brain. The pineal gland is about the size of a grain of rice and shaped like a pinecone (that's how it got its name). One of the principle roles of melatonin is to assist in the regulation of our circadian rhythms, which includes the sleep-awake cycle. Every time it starts to get dark the serotonin levels in your body rise and produce melatonin, which causes drowsiness and a lowering of body temperature in preparation for sleep. Melatonin is also an antioxidant that helps slow down the aging process.

Serotonin deficiency is now known to have some serious side effects including insomnia, chronic anxiety, fatigue, mood swings and strong sugar cravings. The causes? Stress, lack of sleep (talk about a feedback loop!), vitamin and mineral deficiencies, exposure to pesticides in foods and the environment, over consumption of alcohol and caffeine, just to name a few.

On top of that, most people are subject to light pollution and the over-use of artificially produced light. We can make our surroundings appear as daylight when it's the middle of the night. As a result, we don't feel sleepy when we should. We finally fall asleep from exhaustion, and the sleep of exhaustion is not as restful or healing as naturally induced sleep.

I don't mean to get all hippie on you, but moving away from the natural rhythms of nature to which our bodies and internal systems are deeply aligned is not doing us any favors. I'm not suggesting we go back to candles. But I am suggesting we consider how disconnected we've become from our amazing planet and what it's doing to our bodies.

I recently interviewed Octavio Salvado, our yoga instructor in Bali, for my iTunes Channel, *The Happiness Class*. (You'd never guess with a name like that, but he's 100 percent Aussie!) At the end of the interview I asked him to give his top three tips for happiness. He talked about connecting to the natural cycles of each day, and the very first tip he gave was to rise with the morning sun and draw on its rejuvenating and regenerating power. No wonder there is a series of postures in yoga called 'salute to the sun!'

The more connected we are with the planet through the food we eat, the way we sleep, the time we rise, the mindfulness we have when in nature, the healthier we become both physically and mentally.

CHAPTER 28:

Getting into
the Micro and Macro

Resting is not just about going to sleep at night or, if you're a night-worker, during the day. (If you do night shifts, I take my hat off to you. I did it when I was in the military and it's not for the faint of heart. It definitely screws around with your body rhythms.)

Rest means rest—which means taking a break from *doing stuff*. Rest includes taking power naps and breaks. And when I talk about breaks I use the term *micro breaks* and *macro breaks*. Micro means small and macro means large— but I imagine you already figured that out.

Micro Breaks

Numerous studies show that taking regular breaks throughout the day increases performance. One of the best books that goes into breaks at a deep level is *The Power of Full Engagement* by Jim Loehr and Tony Schwartz. In it they cite a study investigating what separates top-seeded tennis players from the next tier down. Players were all doing mostly the same stuff. But there was one differing factor. The highest-seeded players were able to reduce their heart rates between each play of the ball. This meant they were giving their heart and body a micro rest in between plays (by maybe 20+ beats per minute). Their hypothesis? The lower-seeded players tired out more quickly because their heart rate remained elevated for the entire match. This meant more energy consumed and no recuperation of the body in between plays.

Other studies show that taking a mini break every couple of hours can add to productivity and energy levels. And what you do in these mini breaks has a significant impact on their effectiveness. If you stretch – good. If you do breathing exercises – great. If you do gratitude exercises – superb. If you talk to a colleague briefly – wonderful. If you look out over nature or take a short walk in nature – fabulous. If you check Facebook – not so good. If you check how many 'likes' you got on your latest post on Pinterest – not so good. If you gossip, complain or criticize with others during a break – worse than not good.

There are effective ways to take a mini break and there are ineffective ways. If you work with focused bursts of concentration for one hour and then take a 10- minute break and repeat this process, you're likely to be more productive than if you work for four hours straight. More importantly your creativity and innovation increase. Taking mini breaks allows you to have the right combination of focus and energy to tap into your creative juices.

Taking regular breaks ensures the opportunity for drinking enough water, eating properly, and resting your mind—all of which are essential for optimum brain function.

The one exception to taking regular breaks, based on my own experience, is when you're in the creative flow. When you're truly in 'the zone,' you lose track of time. You forget to eat and drink because you're completely absorbed in what you're doing. However, at some point you need to come up for air, food and water if you want to continue functioning optimally over the long term.

Daydreaming

In our over-stimulating world there is very little down time, which means we have to consciously help our bodies get the breaks they need for optimum health and longevity. And daydreaming is a great creative relaxer.

Very few people daydream anymore. Instead they're texting, sexting (which actually might qualify as daydreaming), watching *YouTube* clips, playing games on their electronic devices, checking emails, and making phone calls. And yet daydreaming is not only great fun and a super way to pass time, it's relaxing for the mind and it literally helps shape our lives.

When we daydream, our brains go into an *alpha* brainwave state—a slower state than the beta brainwave state when we're alert, active and concentrating. An alpha brainwave state means the brain is more at rest, consuming less energy. It's also the same brainwave state, along with the even slower rhythms of theta brainwaves, that meditators experience. Can you spell h-e-a-l-i-n-g?

The power nap
Taking a power nap during the day is great for your health, vitality and productivity and I can definitely speak on the benefits from personal experience. I generally experience a productivity dip between 2 pm and 4 pm. I frequently will power nap during this time—which is easy for me since I work for myself, mostly from home.

Power naps come in several sizes and are geared towards specific results. A 15-20 minute nap is great for boosting alertness and motor performance. A 30 to 60 minute power nap boosts decision-making skills because it takes you into a space of 'slow-wave' sleep. For creative problem solving get some REM sleep in a 60 to 90 minute nap.

If you're not in a place where you can lie down or lean back, try doing something physical that doesn't require a lot of brain power, like running errands, picking up groceries, or reading a book. Again, getting out in nature is enormously helpful for de-stressing. Studies with children with ADD and ADHD show that hyperactivity decreases or can sometimes even be eliminated by getting the kids playing outside in a park.

Working with your own rhythms

One of the best things you can do for yourself is to determine your daily energy cycles and then work with them rather than forcing yourself to work to the mechanical ticking of a clock. The clock does not take into consideration any human factors—and unfortunately neither do most corporations. Hopefully one day the world will realize we're our own best masters and judges of how to optimize our productivity.

Until then, if you're in a profession where you're locked into clocking in and out, try presenting a plan to a superior to show them how your effectiveness increases if you work to certain rhythms. You never know until you try! Maybe some bosses will be willing to accommodate.

An example of a biorhythm schedule

I'm most productive during the mornings and evenings—from about 7 am until 1 pm (roughly) and then from 4 pm to 7 pm—and I structure my day according to this rhythm. At the end of my morning meditation I map out the key goals I have for the day, organize emails I have to write and sessions I have with clients and any meetings. Once I've done this I do my physical training for the day, which generally takes 30 to 45 minutes.

At this point I tap into the most productive part of my day. (The book *Spark* by John Ratey cites a number of studies where school children performed better on exams after they did aerobic exercise. Most people are the same way.)

Unless I'm writing, which is one of those 'flow' activities where I can go for two to three hours straight, I do 60 minute bursts of productive work, interspersed with mini breaks when I step away from the desk. I might have a small snack (some raw nuts or a piece of fruit), do some stretches, chat with my partner or play with the dog. Usually I have four, one-hour productivity blocks until I reach my less productive part of the day. Then I break for lunch, take an afternoon siesta or do some mindless tasks.

Isn't it interesting that afternoon siestas were (and still are) a part of many cultures, including Spain, Italy, and Greece? It's all about going with the natural flow of the day. Maybe it isn't the most efficient way to produce the greatest output, but having lived in these parts of the world I can't help but think it's a great way for a community to live and enjoy life. Quite often lunches are social occasions as well, which is great for mental and emotional health.

Which brings up the question about what's most important in life, high output or enjoying life and the close company of others? Personally, I think it's about finding the right mix between productivity (preferably working on something that's meaningful for you) and enjoying your life and the company of others. Around 4pm I go back to work until about 7pm, taking a brief break every hour or so, until the dog with her puppy-dog eyes convinces me I need to take her for a walk.

This is how I generally spend my days Monday to Friday. I also work on Saturday until midday, but reserve my Sundays for doing no work at all. Again, my point here is to find out what works best for you.

Macro Breaks

Life is here for us to enjoy. Yes, there is the suffering thing and the challenge thing and the discomfort thing as well. These are unavoidable and part of growth and are essential for us to experience fulfillment in life. But fun and joy have to be mixed in there too, adding some sort of counter balance to all the challenging experiences. And here's where macro breaks come in.

It's vital to consciously choose to do things that allow us to unplug for extended periods of time. The higher the stress we're experiencing, the longer breaks and/or the more frequent breaks we may need.

Different studies suggest many people would rather earn slightly less money but have more time off work. A 4-day workweek is probably the most doable. Yes, it may require you to reduce your spending, own less stuff and arm-wrestle your boss for the opportunity. But is it worth it to spend more time with your friends and family? To take care of yourself? To take up a hobby you are interested in but never had the time for?

Maybe you love your work so much that you want to be there seven days a week. But even then I think there's incredible benefit in taking at least one day off a week, doing nothing but activities that relax you and increase your connection with other people and the environment. With that in mind, and considering your personal stress levels and needs, let's look at the macro break.

Macro break level one

Do you have at least one day where there is no work? Can you stretch that to two days or even three? For artists, small business owners and entrepreneurs, even having one day off a week can seem like too much of a challenge or overindulgence. But I believe, in the long term, one day off a week is essential for sustainability no matter what you're doing.

Macro break level two

Ideally you need to take a longer break every one to three months. It could be a four or five-day-long weekend getaway up to a two-week vacation. The idea is to down tools and step away from the busyness and high intensity of work for an extended period of time to reconnect with yourself, friends, family, the greater community and with mother nature. Life coach Tony Robbins says, "The quality of your life is in direct proportion to the quality of your relationships." And is he ever right! This is recharge the batteries time when you can deepen your life and consistently put energy back into your relationships so they're around for the long term.

Macro break level three

A decent holiday should happen every year. It's the same principal as a break every one to three months, except it may be for a longer period of time. It takes most people up to a week to totally switch off from work and bring their attention back to what's happening around them so they can be totally present for their relationships.

When I'm travelling internationally I really want to do it in a leisurely way that enables me to connect deeply with the cultures and all the people I meet along the way. Why else am I there? Forget the Five Countries in Five Days approach to travel. That's almost more exhausting than just staying at work.

Macro break level four

This might not be for everyone, but I want you to consider what it would be like if you took an extended break from work. Just sit with it for a bit. What would it feel like to take three months or a year and go on an adventure? What would you do? Where would you go?

Would it be a long, leisurely road trip across your country? How about a long trip through Europe? Australia, the USA, or South America, or Africa, or Asia? What about living in a foreign country for a number of months? Years? How about housesitting a villa in Spain for three months as the owners go off on their own adventure? There are websites that list places you can housesit for free in return for watering the plants, taking care of the house and maybe pets.

The Caretakers Gazette at *www.caretaker.org* is one of the best.

What I'm saying is that these days travel doesn't have to cost you a fortune and sabbaticals are not reserved for university professors. If you have children, house swaps are a great bet. And what better example could you possibly set for your kids than an example of conscious freedom and healthy living?

A formula I've found that's doable is working for five years (still taking shorter breaks in the meantime) and then taking a one-year travel break. It requires that I save 15 percent of my salary (or less if I travel in countries that are cheaper) for five years to have the money to travel for one year. What a deal!

There are so many ways to do this and if you're stuck for ideas on how to manage it, come do some work with me and I'll help you figure it out. There is ALWAYS a way.

Monday to Friday itis

Living in a rut is not optimally healthy, and what I'm trying to do here is encourage you to look at how you can live your life to the fullest—however you define that.

The Western Puritan Work Ethic is like a disease. When I worked in Greece for over two years and then in Italy for a year, I noticed that during the week there were lots of opportunities to catch up with people for dinner or a couple of drinks. People did stuff—they socialized throughout the week. Fun wasn't reserved for the weekends. Plus, in Europe, a month is standard vacation every year for people just starting a job. Weeks are added to that as seniority is gained.

In stark contrast, in western countries (USA, Canada, Australia and UK) you're lucky if you get a single week off your first year of work. And in the West people pine for the weekend so they can have some fun. They rarely take breaks during the week, siestas are unheard of, and work seems to be about getting to hump day (Wednesday) and knowing that you're past the halfway mark. Then life focuses on getting to Friday afternoon and begging the boss for an early knock-off. Then finally you're free at last! On Sunday night people dread going back into work on Monday and starting the grind all over again.

Obviously there needs to be a balance between getting shit done and having down time or you end up with extreme situations with stressed-out, debt-laden unhappy workers and national economic challenges. But I encourage you to give the work/play balance some deep thought. What can you do during the week that will give you something to look forward to that will be a lot of fun? Is it catching up with friends for dinner? Taking the family for a walk down by the ocean, lake, river, etcetera? It may require some organizing, but not much — and isn't that half the fun?

Remember, life is for living everyday, not just Saturday and Sunday.

CHAPTER 29:

Meditation rests the body and mind

Meditation is one of the best practices for increasing your health and happiness and I was unsure which section should include the subject. Not surprisingly, taking the integrated approach to health, it's in more than one place. It's very relevant to resting the body and mind, and it's also a powerful tool when it comes to mindfulness and increasing our cognitive functioning.

Meditation is a brilliant micro-rest break and one of the Top 3 Daily Rituals I teach clients to increase their happiness and health. Meditation has been practiced for thousands of years. Now, with modern measuring equipment like functional MRIs and EEGs, a growing number of mainstream medical professionals are recommending it as one of the most effective techniques to change brainwave states, increase wellness, reduce brain activity, build up stress resilience and allow the body to deeply relax.

I highly recommend using meditation during the day as a great tonic and 'reboot' for your system. If you're one of those people with an overactive mind who has trouble getting to sleep, or problems getting into a deeper REM state, it can be a fabulous tool. Meditation calms the mind, taking it out of the active beta state into a more relaxed alpha brainwave state similar to the dreamy state just before you fall asleep. Meditating for just five to 15 minutes before you go to sleep is an excellent strategy to improve the quality of your sleep. And I highly recommend adding an additional minute to your nighttime meditation to contemplate five things (and people) you're grateful for in your life.

I'll cover meditation in more detail in the Mindfulness Section and give you directions and resources on how to incorporate meditation into your life. I guarantee it will help you de-stress, enhance the quality of your life and improve your overall level of health.

CHAPTER 30:

Tips to getting a great nights sleep

by Sleep Coach Patty Tucker

Tip 1: Set a regular time to get up and go to bed

This means weekends, too. (Yes, I can hear the moans now.)The actual time you choose doesn't matter that much, but being regular about it does. If you have to be up by a certain time to make it to work five days a week, then that's going to be your time, workdays and weekends. This is a crucial step and really hard for most people—especially since we tend to see 'sleeping-in' on weekends as a huge luxury. But if you were getting enough sleep during the week you wouldn't have to catch up on the weekend spending precious playtime unconscious, would you?

Sleep is definitely a natural process and we need to allow the wisdom of nature to work with us. Regular rhythms are a hallmark of nature. We need to join that dance.

Your intended bedtime should be the same every night so you can be certain you're allowing adequate time for quality sleep. I say 'intended' because you may not be sleepy at the same time every night. Even so, it's absolutely necessary to designate a time when all else will be laid aside and sleep will be the priority. Set an alarm clock or your smart phone to let you know that sleeping time is drawing near.

Tip 2: Create a bedtime ritual

If you have kids, or if you ever were one, you're probably familiar with this idea. At a certain time each evening children are reminded to take a warm bath, get into their PJ's, brush their teeth, read a bedtime story, recite their hopes and give thanks, kiss their loved ones and then turn out the lights.

This is an excellent routine to copy as an adult. The advantages are twofold:

1. The regularity of timing is reinforced. Having a regular sequence of activities that lead up to 'lights out' serves as a signal to your body that sleep is approaching. This triggers your system to begin to reset and get ready for sleep.

2. The relaxing nature of pre-bedtime activities gives you an opportunity to shift gears mentally and emotionally. You disengage from the stressors and daily responsibilities and ease into rest. Relaxing reading, listening to soothing music, a bath, a massage, an intimate hour with a lover—all create a transition from active day to restful night.

Tip 3: Create Your Ideal Sleeping Sanctuary

When you walk into your bedroom at the end of a full day, ready to start your successful sojourn to slumber, you should receive one and only one message: Sleep (OK, sleep and sex – but only these two!) If you walk into your bedroom and see a treadmill, a computer, a TV, a pile of laundry, or a pile of anything other than pillows, your brain is getting mixed messages. It doesn't know what you want or intend.

Move everything out of your bedroom that does not relate to or promote good sleep. Here is what else you need to do:

1. You sleep better if it's dark. And I mean DARK. This may seem obvious, but I'm frequently amazed how many people discount this simple fact. The brain gets one of its biggest clues about when to sleep from the daily

changes in light. Melatonin is only produced when the ambient light begins to fade and can be shut down by as little as seven minutes of light exposure. Streetlights, nightlights, the glow from a computer screen, TV or even the alarm clock can be cutting into your ability to produce adequate melatonin to sleep well.

2. You need silence. When the ears pick up human voices, brain wave patterns shift to alert status taking you out of deep sleep. Quiet can be a challenge in some neighborhoods, but good earplugs can be transformational.

3. Don't fall asleep with the TV on. Move it OUT of your sleep sanctuary. Ideally, do not watch TV at least an hour before going to bed. The last thing you need is a bunch of violent images in your brain as you're trying to move into slumber.

4. Sleep comes most easily when the temperature is falling. That's why it's difficult to sleep on hot summer nights. The ideal temperature range for sleep is between 72 and 58 degrees Fahrenheit (22 to 14 degrees Celsius).

5. Buy the most comfortable bed you can afford. When you spend over 2800 hours a year in bed it's worth the investment.

Tip 4: Avoid caffeine, nicotine, alcohol, and sleep disrupting drugs near bedtime

Caffeine, which is in coffee, tea, soft drinks, energy drinks, chocolate and some pain medications, keeps the brain's alert system turned on. The effects can last up to nine hours. That means a diet cola at three pm can keep you up at midnight.

Nicotine has similar alerting effects. Cigarette smokers can also experience withdrawal symptoms during the night causing restless and broken sleep, especially in the latter half of the night.

Alcohol is perhaps the most common self-medication strategy used by people with trouble falling asleep. This can backfire, though. Alcohol can lead to relaxation and quicker sleep onset, but the sleep that ensues is not the deep sleep you want. Also, your liver has to change alcohol into other safer chemicals before elimination can occur. One of those chemicals has stimulant properties similar to caffeine! This happens about four hours after the alcohol hits your stomach—which might explain why you could have a drink at nine, fall asleep at ten, and suddenly be wide-awake at one am.

Tip 5: Get out of bed if you can't sleep

When trying to reset your sleep patterns (or establish more effective ones), you may find even though you've set the stage and done everything recommended that sleep still doesn't come.

If you find yourself awake and getting upset over it, get out of bed. It doesn't matter if it's the beginning of the night, the middle of the night or an hour before the alarm. Do not teach your brain that it's acceptable to be awake in bed. This whole program is about training the brain to know that bed = sleep. If sleep is obviously not on the horizon, get up. Go to another room and do something quiet and restful until you feel sleepy. Then go back to bed and try again. If you wake up as soon as you get back in bed, then get up again. Repeat until you fall asleep easily.

Best Wishes for Peaceful Sleep
Patty Tucker

CHAPTER 31:

Pillar 4 (Rest) Summary

When it comes to rest, these are the most important points:

1. Aim to get 7.5 hours to 9 hours sleep every night. It might mean going to bed earlier at night and/or getting up earlier in the morning.

2. It is important take mini breaks through the day to increase your creativity and productivity. Make sure the mini breaks are positive activities like taking a walk, doing some conscious breathing, daydreaming, speaking with friends or colleagues, reading a positive book, or stretching your body.

3. It is important to consider and then schedule in macro breaks through the weeks, months and years to allow your body and mind to fully relax, regenerate and rejuvenate.

Optimum Health Strategies

1. Start going to bed and getting up at a time that enables you to get at least 7.5 hours sleep a night.

2. If you're having problems with sleep, seek help. I recommend a sleep coach, a wellness or life coach, a naturopath, or other professional who will not just give a sleeping tablet prescription. You need to understand the root cause of your restlessness and work on that.

3. Take at least one day off where you don't work. Aim for at least part of that

day being technology free. (gasp!)

4. Plan and schedule a 2-3 day getaway each month.

5. Plan a longer (3-7 days) getaway every quarter. If possible, do something that's beneficial for your body, mind and spirit, like going to a wellness retreat or spa.

6. Take annual leave. Unplug. Kick your heels up. Have fun. Unwind. Relax.

Recommended Resources

If light and sound pollution (or your partner's snoring) are keeping you from a good night's rest, try a sleep mask and ear plugs. Technology has brought things a long way. You can find masks online in any shape and color. The tempurpedic ones are extremely comfortable and excellent for a complete blackout. But be aware that foam masks (and foam mattresses) may off-gas VOCs (volatile organic compounds).

Stuffing things in your ears is not healthy for the ear canals. The best bet for earplugs are the silicone wax kind that you place *over* the ear opening rather than inside the ear. And they work far better.

Patty Tucker is a sleep coach and consultant helping clients all over the world find their way to the reliable, refreshing sleep they need to live up to their full potential. A graduate of the Stanford Medical Center's Physician Assistant Program, Patty also holds degrees in physiological psychology and political science. If you would like more information or guidance you can e-mail Patty at: **sleepcoach@sleeprestlive.com**

To give you more R&R ideas, at the end of the book I list retreats and courses that I and my team run. Or just go online and search for retreats or courses that are held in places you'd like to visit and include activities you'd like to learn or practice.

Books

- *The Power of Full Engagement* by Jim Loehr and Tony Schwartz.

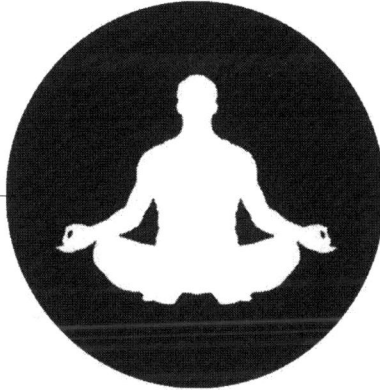

PILLAR 5
MINDFULNESS

All that we are is the result of what we have thought.
Buddha, spiritual leader on whose teachings Buddhism was founded

CHAPTER 32:

Consciousness and the Brain

The human brain/mind connection is ground zero when it comes to optimum health. We've already seen that our thoughts trigger certain related emotions that change the biochemistry and electromagnetic field of the body, affecting our cells and our DNA. Dr. Bruce Lipton, author of *Biology of Belief*, goes so far as to say our cells are like programmable computers responding to their biological environment. And we're the ones doing the programming with everything we think, feel and eat.

This is why this book isn't just about the physical things you can do to optimize your health. Mind is part of the optimum health equation and modern breakthroughs in genetics, epigenetics, brain chemistry, quantum physics and the development of psychiatry and psychology have finally made studying the brain and the mind a legitimate part of health consciousness. So let's get to it!

The Brain 101

Let's get physical. In this section there are three major parts of the brain I'll be talking about:

1. **The Reptilian Brain** — also known as the lizard or hind-brain. It includes the brainstem and cerebellum and was the earliest part of the brain to develop. It controls functions such as heart rate, breathing and body temperature, involuntary and voluntary muscle movement and balance. It also has the highest density of neurons.

2. **The Limbic Brain** — also known as the paleomammalian brain or feeling brain. This is the second oldest part of the brain and the seat of memory formation, emotions, decision-making and the sense of reward, pleasure, and addiction. It allows us to socialize and operate in groups. It also runs the autonomic nervous system and the stress and relaxation response. Neuropeptides, neurotransmitters and hormones are activated via the limbic brain to cause biochemical responses throughout the body otherwise known as feelings. Obviously this is an extremely important part of the brain when it comes to optimum health.

3. **The Cerebral Cortex** — the part of the forebrain or frontal lobe and includes the neocortex. This is the newest, most developed part of the brain responsible for awareness, thought, language and consciousness. It is the part of the brain that processes sensory inputs, coordinates thoughts, actions and internal goals and allows abstract thought and assessment of such concepts as right and wrong. This is the part of our brain that separates homo sapiens from other species on the planet, giving us imagination and the ability to visualize the past and future while living in the present— perhaps our greatest gift and our greatest challenge. I will be referring to the neocortex as the 'thinking' part of the brain.

These three parts of the brain are really not as clear-cut as I've presented them, nor as necessarily specialized. The human brain is still very mysterious. There have been cases of people born with half a brain—or who have suffered brain damage in an accident—who function quite normally because the remaining part of the brain compensates for the missing half. This astonishing ability of the brain to rewire itself is known as neuroplasticity and is very well explained in the book *The Brain That Changes Itself* by Dr. Norman Doidge.

Given neuroplasticity, it is clear our brains are not FIXED. They are malleable and responsive to things we do. I want you to please be 100 percent clear that you're not stuck with a smart or un-smart brain. Whatever you have can be improved upon. It just requires the effective use of one of the brain's functions, the human mind.

The Mind 101

Looking at the intangible mind is harder to do but not impossible given advances in modern research equipment, like a Functional Magnetic Resonance Imaging machine (fMRI) that measures brain activity.

According to some psychological systems, there are three levels of 'mind' — the conscious mind, subconscious mind, and unconscious mind. In some systems of thought the subconscious and unconscious are the same thing. In others they're not. Before we go any further, let's set clear terminology so I don't lose anyone down the rabbit hole.

The conscious mind is information that you're aware of. The word 'awareness' is a good brief definition of the conscious mind. But even this is tricky. We're aware of our environment, both external and internal. We're aware it's raining, that we're driving, that it's hot and that we're hungry and irritated by all the traffic standing in the way of getting to our date at that good Thai restaurant in midtown. But we're actually only dealing with a small amount of the information coming at us.

Our body, with all its senses, sends *11 million bits of information* to the brain per second. Holy cow! You'd think we'd explode with all that input. Which is why all that information is actually compressed down to a consciously manageable level of—you're not going to believe this—around 50 bits of information per second or less to actually consciously process moment to moment.

What happens to all the rest of that information around us? Good question.

The subconscious (called the personal unconscious by Carl Jung) is information you know but are not aware of. The subconscious contains your deepest beliefs and fears and dreams. It contains things that happened when you were a baby or something that happened eight years ago on the second Wednesday in July. You aren't conscious of any of this information. But through hypnosis or some sort of trigger, like looking at a picture, you can make it conscious.

Most of our attitudes, emotions and beliefs are subconscious. For example an early-learned belief that "sex is bad" may run the show when it comes to your intimate relationships and you don't even know it. Things just "never turn out for some reason." You're completely oblivious to what's really going on.

Sensory input that drops below the threshold of conscious awareness—such as background traffic noise or the sound of your refrigerator are part of our subconscious world as well. The sounds are there, but they're subconscious until something makes us aware of them again.

Finally there is the unconscious. Some scientists don't really believe this realm of information exists because it lies 'beyond' all things that are personally knowable or easily relatable or retrievable. The unconscious is the vast, infinite, eternal ocean of information that is the realm of the collective—a boundless, universal mind that transcends the limited separate identity of 'personhood' that is accessible only through deep meditative states of expanded awareness.

The mind and the brain
A lot of people confuse the two, and many scientists believe the mind originates in the brain itself. But the brain is not the mind. The mind is intangible. The mind is consciousness—different levels of information awareness ranging from the highly personal to the vastly impersonal—interacting with the brain. We can't 'see' the mind except as our consciousness interfaces with the brain, actively lighting up different portions of the brain that match the level of consciousness being experienced *through* the brain.

When we're thinking—which most people experience as a verbal 'voice in the head' that follows a linear stream of consciousness—the neocortex is activated and an EEG will record the beta waves of waking consciousness. In someone who is meditating an area of the brain called the anterior cingulate cortex lights up and their brainwave patterns slow into alpha or theta rhythms.

Here lies the gateway to deep relaxation states and the subconscious. There is often no "voice" to this state of consciousness because lower alpha and theta brainwave states are not linear and logical. Here, information processing is more holistic and can be understood more in terms of a deep 'knowingness' about things and an expanded sense of connection, intuition and unity.

When we're in deep sleep and the deepest meditative states tapping into the vastness of the collective unconscious, brainwaves slow down into the delta regions. This is the realm of extreme bliss, 'samadhi,' empathic connectivity with all life or 'oneness' and the realm of many other paranormal experiences.

At the opposite end of the consciousness spectrum from delta there is actually a brainwave state called gamma, which has only recently been discovered, which is faster that beta, reflecting bursts of insight and rapid information processing.

All of these different brainwave states and states of consciousness are related to different areas of the brain. The conscious mind fires up the neocortex. When we're on autopilot and just moving in a habitual fashion, we're more likely to be operating through the reptilian brain. No thought is required. Both the unconscious and subconscious mind (which really kind of blend together), activate the Reptilian and Limbic parts of the brain. Therefore, through the rest of the book, when I refer to the subconscious/unconscious mind, what I'm talking about relates to the physical functions of the Reptilian and Limbic part of the brain.

To put it more simply and keep it general:

- Focused thinking = neocortex (and more specifically the Prefrontal Lobe)
- Automatic pilot = Reptilian and Limbic Brain

However … (I warned you the brain/mind functions are complex!) we can also be on autopilot with our thinking. We all have thought pathways that are well trod—repetitive issues, worries, and fears that are constantly part of our thought processes. They're 'kind of' conscious—we're using the neocortex and thinking, and yet we're unconscious of these repeating patterns of thought

Mindfulness has become a recognizable modern term when it comes to the optimum use of the brain. However, for the rest of this section and the rest of the book, instead of using the term *mindfulness*, I'll be using the term *consciousness*. I believe the more conscious we are of more stuff that's going on inside and outside, the better decisions we make, which subsequently leads to a greater positive impact on our bodies and overall health.

First the bad news

Maybe you think, "Why do I need to learn all this stuff? I'm conscious of what I'm doing!"

I don't like to be the bearer of bad news, but ... once you know this, I promise it will have a positive influence on you. According to science and some of the leaders in the mind-body field like Dr. Bruce Lipton, Dr. Joe Dispenza and Dr. Darren Weissman, humans are generally only conscious of their thinking, feelings and behavior about five percent of the time (plus or minus three percent). This means between 92 to 98 percent of the time, everyone on the planet is running on automatic programs stored in the limbic and reptilian part of the brain—much of which boils down to the fight or flight response.

This answers a lot of questions about the general state of the world, doesn't it? Sure, there are great programs wired into the brain. But there are also a lot of negative programs, like the one that causes you to experience debilitating stress in large social gatherings, or giving a public speech; or the one that makes you panic standing on a high balcony, or facing a very small spider, or the one that puts you into a rage during a disagreement with your partner.

Do we want someone who is highly conscious of their inner processes sitting in a government building with their finger on the Big Red Nuclear Button? Or someone who is not?

Do you want to be as highly conscious of your inner processes so you can be as healthy as possible, or not?

Now the good news

The good news is that past negative programming has an affect on our behavior and physical health only if we remain unconscious of it. Once we become aware of things that trigger inappropriate, unhealthy reactions, we can start working on changing our programming, using our conscious mind to make different choices.

Quantum physics and something called the Observer Effect suggest that once we direct our attention to something we're already affecting a different result. Many people extrapolate this to mean that our attention and intention directly affect things at the quantum level. While this has not been proven scientifically, one thing is certain: when we become aware of limiting thought patterns we can consciously choose another pattern of thought. We can effectively create new neural pathways in our brains and literally rewire how our brains operate.

Our aim is to increase our conscious awareness (that is, increase that five percent figure) and develop programs and associated thinking/feeling habits that put us into a peak and positive emotional state. We want to spend more time in the relaxation response, rather than the stress response.

Sound like a plan?

In the next couple chapters we'll be looking at the things that trip us up and keep us from being more conscious, falling in the same ruts of negativity and ill-health. And we'll be discussing things we can do to create change.

CHAPTER 33:
Things That Keep Us Unconscious

There are many things that stand in line to keep us unconscious—or at least less conscious than we can be. And inertia is one of them.

A body at rest tends to want to stay at rest. It's going to sound ridiculous, but one of the first things we have to do to become more conscious is we have to want to become more conscious. Change takes effort—sometimes a lot of effort. And sometimes it takes some inner coaching to want to even try.

One of the biggest contributors to inertia is the belief we're just fine the way we are. We may feel like crap, but hey, "everybody feels like crap at my age." Bingo. We've just nailed two core-limiting beliefs with one stone.

The topic of beliefs is a big subject. The first digital book I wrote was on beliefs and is 57-pages long; so if you want a deeper dive on the subject, you might want to check out *Your Beliefs are Controlling Your Life*. Right now I will just go into the basics about how beliefs impact our thinking, our feelings, our behavior and the overall health of our bodies.

Subconscious beliefs

Here is what you need to know about beliefs:

1. Most of our beliefs are formed before we are seven years of age. Therefore much of what we believe lies in the subconscious.

2. Prior to age seven we had no ability to discern which beliefs were true, false, good, bad or otherwise. Our brain was doing a constant huge data download of input from the environment so we could become independently capable of survival. But at the same time we had no discernment or even the ability to question the beliefs we were being taught by others. Plus, as children we spent most of our time in a theta or alpha brainwave state — the same states characterizing hypnosis. So we were very open to direct suggestion.

3. Once we were taught a belief (indirectly or directly, verbally or via observation), we unconsciously looked for evidence to support the belief. What you look for you generally find, often at the expense of noticing the opposite may also be true. Beliefs thus become very one-sided. Although we tend to live as though they're universal laws like gravity, most beliefs are not 100 percent 100 percent of the time.

4. Other people's beliefs, even our parents, aren't necessarily valid for our lives or even the day and age we live in.

5. Your life is created by your beliefs. This is great when the beliefs support your best self possible, but sucks when your beliefs cause you to be less than you are capable of being. (Welcome to the world!)

6. Our beliefs determine the meaning we give things in our lives. For instance, if I have a belief that says, "Travelling on airplanes is unsafe," I'm likely to feel scared when I have to take a flight for work or pleasure. The belief gives meaning to the experience of flying, which can be summed up as: flying means danger. This causes my body to initiate a stress response, which deactivates my immune system. However, if I believe flying is safe, then I'm more likely to be relaxed, excited, and physically unaffected by the thought or actuality of flying.

As you can see, our beliefs have a major impact on our lives and our health. Through a higher level of consciousness—by being aware—we notice what beliefs and thoughts we're carrying and which are serving us and which are leading to suffering. Once we attain and maintain conscious awareness, we can choose thoughts and behaviors that better serve us, causing a life-enriching chemical relaxation-response cocktail to course through our bodies.

Lack of wisdom

One of the biggest things tripping us up in our pursuit of greater awareness is lack of wisdom. And what is that anyway?

I want you to picture a wise man or woman. What do they look like? What are they wearing? How are they moving? How are they speaking? How do they deal with situations or challenges? How do they move through life? Do they move slowly or are they in a rush to get things done? (Yes, I'm tipping you towards seeing the same picture as me. But it's a good picture!)

The wise person I see is moving purposefully. They're getting perspective on a situation from many different angles. They're firing up their powerful minds to consider all the consequences to difference choices. Then they're *responding* in a deliberate and thoughtful way, showing a high level of *CONSCIOUSNESS*.

As we know, the more consciousness we bring into our lives, the more aware we are of what's working and not working—especially when it comes to our health. **Our life, and especially our health, is directly related to the sum of the choices we make for good or ill** from moment to moment. The better choices we make, the better results we get. To facilitate this we need to know:

1. What do I need to be aware of?
2. What are the better choices once I know what I'm dealing with?

This entire book is about answering these two questions as they relate to optimum health. Knowing the answers, then acting on the information and having the experience of optimum health as a result of what you learn here adds up to what I define as WISDOM: the sum of our knowledge and our experiences in any given area.

Maybe it would be nice to have a crystal ball and see into the future. But the wise man and wise women doesn't need one. For them, the best guarantee of a happy life is based on making the best decisions based on the most current information and the likely consequences of various actions based on their past experience. It's not an infallible formula, but it does lead to the likelihood of better results.

Here are a few ways to increase WISDOM in any particular area:

Increase Knowledge:
1. Read non-fiction books, autobiographies, and blogs to broaden your understanding of different subjects.
2. Listen to talks, presentations, seminars, and recordings presented by teachers you respect.
3. Undertake formal study through online courses or a physical institution or training establishment. The great thing these days is you don't need to spend four years learning a new profession.
4. Ask questions and listen intently to a person who has done something you want to do so you understand how they achieved it. Draw on their wisdom to increase your own. Look for mentors.

Increase Experience:
1. Step out of your comfort zone (also called the 'known'). Try new things. Attempt something you haven't done before. Push against physical, mental or emotional resistance in order to grow and understand at a deeper level.
2. Find someone doing what you would like to do and follow him or her. Ask them to mentor you, or hire a coach to show you, experientially, how to do

something and then go experience it while under their guidance.

3. Be bold, courageous, spontaneous, curious, and open to new experiences that present themselves.

My final point on wisdom is that increasing wisdom through knowledge and action is actually the same thing as rewiring the brain. *Hebb's Rule* (named after Donald Hebb, a psychologist known most prominently for cell assembly theory) says "Neurons that fire together, wire together." Which means if we fire up our conscious mind and make a study of something, it causes a physical neural response in the brain, creating new neural pathways. That is why we are not 'fixed' with a set level of intelligence or ability. Our brains, through repetition of a new thought, feeling or behavior and the firing of the associated neurons, can build entirely new patterns.

For example, in a study performed by Sara Lazar at the Psychiatric Neuroimaging Research Program at Massachusetts General Hospital, she found that the parts of the brain involved in self-reflection and empathy were significantly thicker in meditators than in controls who did not meditate.

The opposite of *Hebb's Rule* is also true. Parts of our brain can also atrophy (degenerate) if they're not used – neurons that don't fire together, don't wire together. So, just as we have to continue to use our muscles against an appropriate source of resistance to keep them strong, we also need to keep challenging our minds to keep both mind and brain healthy and functional.

Knowledge + experience = Wisdom = new mind = new you!!

I can just see that five percent level of consciousness expanding now!

Runaway thinking and emotions

In a very general sense, positive emotions are good for our physical health and negative emotions, if they persist, are detrimental to our health. It's okay to feel those 'negative' emotions like fear, worry, anger, frustration, disconnection, sadness, etcetera. They're a normal part of life for a human being. Issues occur if the negative emotions persist for extended periods of time.

The stress of continuous negative emotions and constant activation of the stress response can cause the body to break down because the body needs to be in the relaxation response to self-regulate and self-heal. And who hasn't sometimes felt like they were caught on a hamster wheel when it comes to some painful thought process or emotion?

"I just can't help feeling angry all the time," says a friend. We can all relate.

Unfortunately, if we follow *Hebbs Rule*, this means that the more anger we feel in more and more situations the bigger our brain's neuronal pathways for anger get. Pretty soon, if we don't watch out and become conscious of what's going on, most of the thoughts we have end up being related to anger. This burns out the adrenal glands and makes it difficult for the brain's neurons to be able to accept other neurotransmitters except those related to anger.

In most cases, our thinking triggers our emotions. The exception is when our limbic brain is triggered prior to us consciously assessing a particular situation. Take the example of going on a trek through a forest and reacting to what appears to be a snake. Your body automatically goes into the stress response. Once the conscious mind gets into gear you realize the 'snake' is actually a stick. Then you consciously wind your body down, return your breathing and heart rate to normal, and get back to relaxing and enjoying the gorgeous scenery around you.

The thing is, when you're in a tape loop with negative thoughts and emotions running, you're more susceptible to limbic triggers. With the body in a constant stress response, it's hard to see things clearly—whether it's a stick or a difficult client at work that always seems to push your buttons.

The more conscious we become the less easily we get caught in these kinds of cycles. But the first step is realizing that none of us is perfect and that we're not at the mercy of our emotions. (Part one of gaining wisdom.) Only then do we have the motivation to learn all the ways we can handle and change our emotions and the thoughts that cause them. (Part two of gaining wisdom.)

We'll talk about methods of changing and increasing consciousness in the next chapter.

CHAPTER 34:

Consciousness in daily life

Now we move from theory to practice. Theory is not worth a pinch of salt if it's not followed up with practical application. If there are two people and the first person has read 100 books but has not applied one thing, and the second person has read one book and taken specific action even on one point, the second person is likely be out in front.

So how do we live a more conscious life? How do we increase our overall level of consciousness?

One of the greatest things we can do to immediately increase our level of consciousness is SLOW DOWN. When we slow down, we can be more deliberate about where we direct our attention. We have the space to notice what our bodies are telling us moment to moment about our health. We notice what feelings we're generating, whether it's joy, fear, happiness, anger, frustration, excitement, etc. When we slow down and become more conscious, we have the ability to consider the consequences of the actions we're about to take. We can better decide where we're going physically, the words we speak, the beliefs we buy into, and the foods we put into our bodies.

Remember that wise man or woman we were talking about in the last chapter? The wise person moves slowly—not slowly physically (though they might at times) but rather they move deliberately. They respond to situations rather than *reacting* to life.

Acting like a wise person of heightened consciousness looks like this:

1. Something happens, you're asked something, or someone says or does something to you (called an Event).
2. You pause or stop.
3. You breathe and connect to your senses and feelings.
4. If you sense a reactive emotion like anger or fear, notice it but don't buy into it. Breathe slowly and deliberately and consciously calm the body down.
5. 'Step back' and observe yourself and the situation to gain a broader perspective.
6. Think about information and experiences pertinent to the situation with a focused, conscious mind.
7. You decide.
8. You deliberately act on your decision.

Slowing down is a life changer. The slowing down does not necessarily have to be physical—though I suggest sometimes doing things deliberately and consciously (which may appear slower) can produce a better result. The idea is to bring a high level of consciousness to whatever you're doing.

Imagine cruising along at a leisurely pace as opposed to scrabbling around, rushing, racing, backtracking and bouncing off walls. Just imagining 'normal' modern chaos gives me a mild stress response! So if slowing down is so good for us and makes sense intellectually, then why don't we all do it?

Well, remember, we're generally only conscious about five percent of the time and the rest of the time we're on autopilot—being run by programs and beliefs we've picked up over the course of our lives. Some of them are genetic, but most of the influential programs are learned beliefs and behaviors we picked up in our formative years. Here are a few typical programs about speed:

• I must do this quickly otherwise I will miss the opportunity. (Get it while the getting's good.)

- I'm not worthy of health and happiness unless I work harder and faster than everyone else.
- If I finish first I am a winner. When I win I feel significant and loved. (This is common and probably the result of a parent or parents showing more affection to their child when they won something. It also leaves a deeper belief that not winning means less significance and less love.)
- I have to achieve all of this right now to prove I'm a good employee/mother/wife/husband/father etc. (The expectations are generally self imposed and again the result of a deeper program which suggests something like: If I don't achieve enough (X) I am UNWORTHY of love.)

Because of these kinds of subconscious beliefs, when we do try to slow down the stress response kicks in and we feel a general discomfort in our bodies. We think at some level that slowing down is wrong and will stop us from achieving what we want in life. There is no physical threat, just a *psychological* threat.

Slowing down is vital for tuning into our bodies and emotions, getting clarity about what we feel, what we want to feel, what we want to have and do, and for formulating the most effective plans for getting those things. It really helps to understand what beliefs may be stopping us from slowing down. A good way to find out is to do the following sentence completion exercise, which I suggest you do either now or when you come to the end of the chapter. (What's stopping you from doing it right now? Are you in a hurry to get to the end of the chapter? ;-)

This exercise could be a huge ah-hah moment for you and a course correction for your health and happiness, so take your time and finish the following sentences with at least 10-20 responses. The more responses you write, the deeper you are getting into uncovering your subconscious beliefs.

- When I slow down it makes me feel...
- When I slow down I think it will...

(Or another way of phrasing it is:)

• When I slow down I think _____ (fill in the blank) will happen.

After you've written your answers, ask yourself where these beliefs came from. Ask yourself, "Do these beliefs serve me? Are they really true or are they something I've taught myself to believe? Would I be better off without them? How would having an opposite or different belief change my life?"

By the way, if you don't have any issues with slowing down and you find it easy to stop, think and deliberately act, then I am giving you a round of applause. Well done!

Finally, slowing down gives you the time to create the vision of what it is you want to achieve in life. What are your short-term goals? Long-term goals? What do you want the end results to look like? The more time you take addressing your vision of what you want in life, the clearer you become and the better the results are likely to be.

A wee look at your vision

A higher level of consciousness includes choosing your vision(s), selecting the feelings you would like to experience and determining the behaviors that are most in alignment those feelings. It's also about becoming aware of the thoughts, feelings and behaviors that are not conducive to the successful expression of the vision and then replacing them with the thoughts, feelings and behaviors that are. Obviously one of your visions is optimum health, radiance, vitality, and youthfulness or you wouldn't be reading this book!

So, where the heck does vision come from? **How do we know if it is a *good* vision, one that will lead us down the right path?** Here are the essential keys to finding the 'right' vision.

1. The vision needs to be in alignment with your personal values, personal strengths, desires, needs and personal feelings. Don't borrow someone else's vision (regardless of how persistently they try to ram it down your throat). Own your own vision.

2. Just as you have your own unique fingerprint amongst 7 billion people, you also are like no one else on the planet. Your vision needs to be about fully expressing your uniqueness. If a vision requires you to be or act like someone else, then it's not your vision.

3. Your vision does not have to be about saving the world, your country, your city, community or even your family. It's more important to have a vision that allows you to be you. And here's the thing: when you have a vision that allows you to be you, you're making the world a better place. Imagine a world with more authentic people. How good would that be?

4. Your specific vision(s) may change over time. In fact, if the circumstances around you change, or you feel a need to change, then review your vision and change it if necessary. Your vision is more like a guiding star than a rulebook.

5. The right vision lights you up. It feels right. It clicks like a key fitting into a lock. You have a deep sense of "YEAH! This is for me! This is me!"

6. The right vision taps into your strengths, causes you to feel the feelings that are most important to you, causes you to grow, and increases your level of consciousness. But it is not necessarily easy or free of challenge, because the right vision, by its very nature, is there to make you grow into the fullest expression of yourself.

7. Vision demands change. Often we need to leave things behind, or stop doing things, or start doing things, or push against resistance, or face our fears, or change course, or step out of our comfort zone, or start again. None of these things are easy. But they just might be what is needed for you to fully express yourself.

Vision, choice, perspective and integrity

Without perspective it's hard to make good choices about anything, let alone your vision. You need to be very aware of where you are now, where you want to end up and what the possible ways to get there are. Observation is something you need to do on a regular basis. Are you on track with your vision? Observe how you feel. Does it still feel right for you? Or has something changed along the way that you need to make necessary adjustments for?

What do you really want?

This is a tough one, and very similar to your vision being in alignment with your personal beliefs, strengths and values.

Sometimes we don't even know a choice is not ours. Maybe you believe you really really want to be a lawyer. But when you're finally practicing law you really dislike it and stress to the point of chronic fatigue or similar health issues. You thought you'd like it, but when you reflect back on your life you realize the idea was IMPLANTED in your mind by your parents, or a teacher, or a particular life event.

This is where you need to dig deep. Before you make any choice and before you set any vision in motion ask yourself if what you *think* you want is the same as what you *feel* you want. **What is your heart telling you?** What is your gut telling you? What feels right? This is the time to get out of your head and get into your heart, because that's where what you really want is hanging out.

Who do you want to be?

How do you want to be remembered on the epitaph of your gravestone? You want to make choices and create visions that allow you to express the person you deeply want to be. If there's a safe choice that doesn't allow you to be who you know you need to be, then you might need to kick that choice out the door and go for something that allows you to be courageous, daring and an adventurer. Choose who you want to be, then make choices that allow you to be that person.

How do you want to feel?

This is a biggy. Figuring out the core feelings you want to experience and then setting the goals and visions and making choices that will allow you to feel these feelings is a huge part of making choices and creating your vision. There are some great books written about this process. One book I recommend is *The Fire Starter* by Danielle LaPorte.

Who is affected?

Part of functioning at a high level of consciousness is also about being aware of who and what may be affected by your decisions. Will your friends and family be affected in a positive way? Will your choices positively impact you and your health? Will your choice be good for the community outside of your inner circle? Will this choice be good for the environment and the planet you live on?

Integrity

Everything we just discussed is really about integrity. Being a conscious decision-maker and a higher conscious human being means what you're doing, choosing, thinking, saying, and feeling is aligned with your highest vision for yourself and the world. This is integrity.

What are you telling yourself?

What do you tell yourself as you move through your day? Is your internal dialogue positive or negative? Are you telling yourself you *can* or you *can't*? Are you criticizing yourself, or are you compassionate with yourself?

We believe the voice inside our heads and even think we are the internal dialogue. That is, we believe the essence of who we are is the speaker inside our head. Often our internal dialogue happens beneath our conscious awareness. And often it's been playing the same song for decades. The reality is, the internal monkey chatter in our minds is no more 'us' than the external chatter at a social gathering. There may be some worthwhile inner dialogue, but mostly it's a lot of crap.

The thing to realize is we are not the dialogue; we are the observer of the dialogue. Therefore we can choose which conversations we want to be a part of and which ones we need to evict from the party in our minds.

The way to deal with the internal dialogue is to see it for what it mostly is — noise. Choose what statements to listen to, which ones to expand upon, which ones are the best ones to influence your decisions and vision and which ones to kick to the curb. You can choose a new dialogue. You can start a new conversation. You can make a bold new statement. You just need to say it enough, connect with it emotionally, see it, feel it, and experience it to effectively rewire your brain to be your best support, not your worst inner critic.

What language are you speaking?

This section isn't about dialect; it's about the words you're speaking and the tone of your speech. It's about what you're creating in the physical world as a result of the words that are leaving your lips.

Neuro-Linguistic Programming (NLP) is a personal development methodology created in California in the 1970s by Richard Bandler and John Grinder. Its premise is that language and behavioral patterns are neurological processes that can be changed to facilitate specific goals in life.

As an NLP Master Practitioner I am very conscious of the words I use and the words and language used by my clients. The words, phrases and sentences that we use can make us feel good or bad. They can empower us or disempower us. They can make others feel better or feel worse. They can cause us to go into a stress response. They can direct and misdirect our attention. They can also cause us to feel a particular emotion.

The words we speak originate in our brains, and they can either come from a place of consciousness (where words are selectively chosen) or they can come from a loop recording of an old unconscious pattern which may or may not serve us in a good way. Words are the physical expression of our thinking put out into the world. They are one of the ways we let people know who we are.

To help you discover the power of words I want you to read through the following statements. You can read them silently or aloud:

1. I was stabbed in the back by one of my friends.

2. This always happens to me.

3. I am always struggling with my health.

4. I hate it when there is a line at the cinema.

5. I should visit my brother more often.

6. I can't do it.

Now, let's put our NLP caps on and have a closer look at these sentences to see if they are empowering or disempowering (relaxing or stressing).

1. Were you really stabbed in the back? Or did someone say something you didn't like or felt was mean or thoughtless? The emotions associated with being physically stabbed in the back are a lot more intense (and potentially damaging to the body) than the emotions of someone saying something you didn't like.

2. Does this always happen to you? Really? Or has it happened a few times? Or a lot? When we exaggerate we actually create more intense emotions.

Great if we're always having great stuff happening. Not so great if we're getting hyper-focused on a negative situation that, most likely, does not 'always' happen. Negative exaggeration affects our health negatively.

3. Always struggling. As with #2, 'always' implies 24/7 and is pretty horrific to imagine. It also can become a self-fulfilling prophecy. I call using words like 'always' as speaking in absolutes. There is no room to move. It eliminates any possibility of something else occurring. 'Struggling' is also a fairly graphic, emotional word that is more applicable when we're talking about wrestling pythons or lions.

4. Hate. This is an intense word and again creates a strong emotional (and biochemical) response in the body. Do you 'hate' something or is it mildly bothersome? Your body (and cells) experience two very different reactions between 'hate' and 'bothersome.' Tone it down wherever possible.

5. I should... I am actually a big fan of dumping the 'should' word from the English language (I'm not sure if there is an equivalent word in other languages). Albert Ellis, one of the top psychologists of the last century, also had a major problem with the 'should' and 'must' words. The problem with these words is they remove our autonomy and choice and imply that something outside of us knows better. When I hear someone say, "I should..." I say: "Who or what says you should? Why should you? What will happen if you don't? What do you CHOOSE to do, based on your knowledge, experience and the current reality?" A basic human need is the feeling we have autonomy and some control over our lives. When we 'should' on ourselves, we're handing over our choice to something or someone else.

6. I can't. Hmmm. Have you just closed the door on possibility? The word 'can't' is a show-stopper. Now you have no choice and no chance! Remember, even our brains are malleable. With guidance, focus, practice, repetition and persistence we can change most things. The 'can't' will become a 'not yet,' which will eventually become a 'can.' Always replace can't with 'not yet.'

The more we focus on the negative the more negative stuff happens. We stop noticing the good and draw our attention to the bad while just to the left or right of our vision may be a garden full of roses.

I challenge you, right now, to pay 100 percent attention to the language you use for the rest of the day and then the rest of this week. This is one of the activities I always set for my clients. I also suggest that they pay particular attention to the language other people use around them.

Are they using positive words and sentences or are they using language that is negative and critical? Pay attention to how your words and other peoples' words make you feel. Do the words make you feel better or worse? Do they make you feel more capable or less capable? Do they help you to relax or do they create stress? Do they inspire you or expire you? Know, beyond a shadow of a doubt, that your words and the emotions they evoke affect your health for better or worse.

Authentic emotions

Managing (and processing) your emotions is a key to optimum health and happiness. One of the principle ways to maintain high consciousness is to fully feel your emotions. Don't suppress them and don't wallow in them. Feel them and observe them to discover what they're trying to tell you. This is being conscious of your emotions and the messages they're sending you.

Have you ever traveled to Thailand? It's a beautiful place, full of beautiful people. And much of the culture is about smiling, being softly spoken, saying 'thank you,' being nice to others and not offending people.

When talking recently to a colleague who lives in Thailand, he mentioned how a number of Westerners had been shot or beaten up by Thai people when they verbally expressed their anger at the Thai person. Now, if verbal criticism, even if expressed angrily, provokes someone to the point where they beat up another person or kill them, this is a red flag revealing there are *suppressed* and *unprocessed* emotions lurking in the shadows.

I'm always interested to see if the external persona someone projects matches their internal emotional condition. Are they calm on the outside as well as on the inside where it really matters? Or are they being inauthentic?

A person who feels anger but suppresses it to put on their 'happy' face does not do their psychology or health any favors. On the other hand, the person who feels angry, expresses it appropriately, comes to fully understand why they're angry and accepts themselves, is much better off. It's not just about the negative emotions; it's about what we *do* with them. Do we learn from them? Do we feel them fully? Do we accept ourselves even though we have them? Do we process them? Do we understand what they're telling us and then do we do something about them?

To feel angry is okay. To get stuck in anger is not okay. To feel sad is normal. To feel sad and continue on a downward spiral until you get sick is obviously not healthy. Emotions need to be acknowledged by being felt so they can be understood and processed.

If you stick with an emotion, truly seeing it, feeling it and hearing what it has to say, it will move through you and be resolved. There's a great book on the *Emotional Freedom Technique (also called 'tapping')* by Nick Ortner called *The Tapping Solution*. I highly recommend it for processing emotions. Part of the physical technique involves verbally acknowledging that you accept yourself no matter what you're feeling. And this is the perfect starting step to processing negative emotions.

Acceptance means realizing there is nothing wrong with you no matter what you're feeling. You're still worthy of being loved and having a place on planet

Earth. In the next section on wholeheartedness I will share a great technique for processing emotions taught by Dr. Darren Weissman in his book *The Heart of the Matter.*

Compassion

Are you showing a high level of compassion for yourself in your daily life? Are you being compassionate with other people? Or are you being overly judgmental?

Compassion has been the focus of numerous spiritual and religious practices over the millennium because it's one of the most powerful healing emotions and one of the most powerful expressions of love. Compassion definitely requires a conscious shift out of your head and into your heart and feeling nature, which is what enables you to 'tune in' to your own needs and the needs of others.

It definitely takes practice moving out of judgment into a more allowing space.

Are you hard on yourself or other people about something? What exactly? What are the issues that make you hard and tough and inflexible? Contemplate what it would look like bringing more compassion into your life, first for yourself, then others.

The more connected you are with your heart, the less you will experience the kind of shutting-down, loneliness and the negative health issues associated with isolation and disconnection.

Over-stimulation of the brain

Hands up if you are using 100 percent of your potential?

My hand is definitely not up! We all know we have more potential than we're using, but we also recognize there's a limit to what we can handle in a healthy way. Over a certain level of demand I think we start going backwards. Regardless of potential we have individual capacities when it comes to handling the competing demands for our attention.

Do you have the consciousness to know when you're being healthily pushed? Can you tell when you're about to explode? Be kind to yourself. Tune in to where you're at as far as tolerating busy-ness is concerned. At a certain point (and only you know what that point is) you have to start saying 'no' to additional commitments.

The conscious mind has limits. When there is too much distraction and environmental stimuli, the effort of processing the external stimuli to determine if there are potential threats fatigues the mind. The constant switching of focus and the redirection of attention is very draining work for the brain and consumes a lot of energy.

How many things do you have in your life that bleep, buzz, tweet, ping, beep, ring, tap, and vibrate? How many things are constantly drawing your attention away from one thing and onto another? As you are doing one task, how many times are you pulled away by a beep on your Smartphone?

The idea that multi-tasking is a good thing is not supported by any research. In the book, *Your Brain At Work*, David Rock sites numerous studies reinforcing the idea that brains function best when they have a single point of focus. Some people may think they're great at multi-tasking, but the reality is, each individual task would have a better result if it were the single point of your focus.

The most successful people on the planet have the ability to laser-focus their attention on a particular task to the exclusion of all distraction. It's this single-pointedness that produces magical works of art, incredible music, world records, and billion-dollar businesses.

So, consider the distractions you have in your life.

Apply your vision and decision-making skills and choose the ones that are most important and sideline the rest. And here's another consciousness-raising tip: I truly believe one of the best detoxing activities we can incorporate into our lives is to unplug ourselves from technology on a regular basis for short periods of time (and even extended periods of time). Who hasn't felt stressed when they're on their way somewhere and realized they've forgotten their cellphone, only to feel greatly relaxed later on, after doing without it for the day?

Ahhh, what bliss.

CHAPTER 35:

Meditation

There is an incredible volume of research and material available on meditation, and a matching amount of interest in the medical and scientific community on its positive effects. Even the Dalai Lama encourages long-term meditating monks to participate in scientific research. The overall conclusion? Meditation has amazing benefits for both the body and mind. I've been meditating daily anywhere from 15 minutes to an hour for the last four years (at the time of this writing) and meditation is one of the Top 3 Daily Rituals I recommend everyone adopt (along with physical activity and a Green Drink) to get the very best out of themselves.

Why meditation is so great

The body cannot perform at its optimum and self correct if it's not given the opportunity to do so. It's like an engine running at full capacity non-stop. It will eventually wear down without downtime and maintenance. Meditation is just the thing to balance out our fast-paced lives.

Cardiologist Dr. Herbert Benson, author of *The Relaxation Revolution*, has studied and written about meditation for decades, actually coining the term *relaxation response*—which is exactly what meditation induces in our bodies. According to Benson, the relaxation response is characterized by the following physiological responses: decreased metabolism and muscle tension, decreased oxygen consumption, heart rate, blood pressure and rate of breathing; a calming in brain activity, an increase in attention and decision-making functions of the brain, and changes in gene activity.

Can you spell 'good for you?'

Some of these effects are associated with sleep as well. But where it might take hours to experience these effects via sleep, with meditation it takes only minutes for the body to wind down and start doing the necessary self-healing work. Not only do you get the benefits of sleep more quickly, meditation is more active than sleep. You actively focus your attention in meditation, which makes it like a workout for the brain.

Matthieu Ricard, author of *Why Meditate* says, "Over the course of the last ten years, I have participated in several research programs intended to document the long-term effects of meditation practice on the brain and on behavior. This research has shown that it's possible to make significant progress in developing qualities such as attention, emotional balance, altruism, and inner peace. Other studies have also demonstrated the benefits of meditating for 20 minutes a day. These benefits include a decrease in anxiety, a decrease in vulnerability to pain, a decrease in depression and anger, as well as strengthening the power of attention, boosting the immune system, and increasing one's general well being. No matter what point of view you approach it from—whether that of personal transformation, the development of altruistic love, or physical health—meditation emerges as a factor essential for leading a balanced life, rich in meaning."

Another reason why meditation is so good for us is it positively affects the expression of the genes in our DNA. "In the long-term practitioners [of meditation], the genes that controlled metabolism, stress, aging of the body were activated," says Benson. "Genes that were controlling the immune system and inflammation systems of the body were quieted down. There was little change in the control group. With this finding there could no longer be any separation between mind and body. The mind could quiet the body at the genetic level."

Meditation studies by Sara Lazar, PhD, of the MGH Psychiatric Neuroimaging Research Program, found increased grey-matter density in the hippocampus of meditators (a brain area known to be important for learning and memory), and in structures associated with self-awareness, compassion and introspection. Participants also reported reductions in stress.

Bottom line, meditation shows us we have a lot more control of our consciousness and health than we're lead to believe!

The 'how to'

ALL the thoughts we have are about the past or future.

Thinking about that statement you're already in the past, dwelling on a moment gone by. If you're truly present, in the now, you aren't thinking, you're just feeling the moment, experiencing what you're experiencing. It really is a peaceful place to be. Interestingly enough, the past/present nature of our thoughts is stressful to the body. They're literally telling the body it needs to be somewhere else and some *when* else in time.

When you bring your attention into the present moment to feel the breeze on your skin, or the smell of the air before a storm, or lose yourself in the brightness of the colors around you, you feel relaxed and connected. As far as 'doing' meditation is concerned, it's less about doing and more about increasing the gap between your thoughts and hanging out in the nothingness (thoughtless) zone, simply being, as long as possible.

Let me start off with the basic physical practice and then I'll answer some common questions people ask. Here are the basics of how to meditate:

The Setting

1. Find somewhere quiet where you won't be disturbed and where the light

isn't too bright. Do NOT take your cell phone with you!

2. Sit rather than lay down, as you are less likely to fall asleep.

3. Maintain a straight posture without being too rigid. You don't want to lean backwards or forwards, just comfortably with minimal back arch.

4. I recommend practices where the eyes are closed. There are different practices where the eyes are left open, but they require some coaching. By closing your eyes you're reducing a lot of brain activity associated with visional stimulation and mental visual.

5. Sit in the same place every day if possible. This will create an association with the physical space and cause the brain and body to automatically start moving into a deeper relaxed state as soon as you sit down.

6. The best times to meditate are soon after waking and before going to bed, as your brainwave activity is already likely to be reduced to a low beta or high alpha brainwave state at these times. The next best time is whatever time you can do it. It's FAR more important you do it than wait for the 'perfect' time.

The 'doing'

1. Relax your belly and focus on breathing deeply and fully — and that means with your diaphragm. Your stomach will move with the inhalations and exhalations.

2. Focus on your breathing. This is one of the most simple and effective ways to relax your mind and body. If you can, breath in and out of your nose. Connecting to your breath is connecting to life – literally. Because if you disconnect from breathing for more than a few minutes you stop being connected to life permanently.

3. You can place your hands in a number of different positions. The most popular is with the thumb and index finger touching while the back of the hands rest on or near the knees.

4. When thoughts come, (and they will!) let them pass you by without directing your attention to them. Simply watch your breath.

5. For many of us, sitting in a cross-legged posture (like you would see ancient and modern yogis or monks doing) is uncomfortable. However, if you put a pillow under your butt, it changes the positioning of your hips enough to make it more comfortable. If you can't sit cross-legged, then sitting in a chair is perfectly fine.

How long should I meditate?

There are a number of different opinions about this. Dr. Benson says between 10-20 minutes is sufficient to create the relaxation response. Most teachers say around 15 minutes is enough to experience the major benefits from meditation. Some sources suggest twice a day for about 20 minutes. Of course, if you really want to make significant changes to your emotional and psychological wellbeing, you can meditate for 1-2 hours at a stretch, or longer if you're so inclined.

From my personal experience and reading, I suggest that you aim to get to a point where you're meditating for **about 15 minutes every day**. Sometimes you might do more and sometimes less, depending on the circumstances. There are times when 40 minutes fly by, and others where eight minutes is a stretch.

If you are new to meditating, take my advice and don't sweat the length of the meditation. Doing it is what counts. It might only be three minutes. The most important thing as a beginner is *getting in the habit of showing up*. You want to create a habit of sitting down to meditate. Extend your practice to 15 minutes over time, but be prepared for this to take several weeks to achieve on a daily basis.

Am I doing it right?

One of the first things is to suspend all judgment about whether you are doing it 'right.' The aim is to have no judgment about your meditation. Just do it because it's great for you. Forget trying to figure out whether your meditation was Zen-like or not. You just can't judge. You might think your meditation session was all over the place, but the actual brainwave activity might show great symmetry between the two hemispheres of the brain. It's safe to assume all meditation is good meditation.

Also, I've had clients who have been meditating for a whole week say to me, "I can't understand why I still have these random thoughts popping up in my mind." Welcome to Meditation 101. Rome was definitely not built in a day or even a year or even five years—and neither is the creation of a 'still' mind. It takes as long as it takes for the monkey chatter in your mind to calm down and dissipate.

Remember. It's not so much about the thoughts that pop into our mind—it's about what we focus our attention on. In meditation you're aiming to focus on your breath and the space between your thoughts, holding your attention on the emptiness. When an unannounced thought pops up and you are drawn to it, notice you are being drawn, say "oh, well," and then take your attention back to your breath.

Useful Resources

Most quality yoga classes start and end with meditation and breathing exercises, so yoga classes are a great way to learn meditation. You also might want to check out some meditation classes to get a better idea of the tips and strategies to help you with your practice. There are many different kinds.

Several years ago when I committed to doing a 365-days-a-year meditation practice, I realized I needed help and ended up purchasing some guided meditation audio recordings (MP3s), which I still use occasionally. I have a number of guided meditation recordings that range from 14 minutes to one hour. Some have background sounds like waterfalls, rain, Tibetan bells or the like. CDs are extremely useful if you live somewhere that is noisy or you live in a house in Bali that is designed to let in the outside environment along with the next-door neighbors' kids doing *School of Rock* practice.

There is also new audio technology available which assists you in attaining deeper brainwave states through subliminal sounds. Essentially the sounds are at different frequencies outside the range of our normal hearing. I have definitely been able to go much deeper in a meditation when I used a meditation CD recorded with subliminal audio technology. One my favorite organizations in the wellness industry is *The Entheos Academy* (spear-headed by the very cool Brian Johnson) and they have a line of guided meditation resources called *Blissitations* – so check them out.

A final word on meditation

Here is a final quote from Jon Kabat Zinn, Ph.D, author of *Wherever You Go There You Are* and a meditation teacher who is passionate about bringing mindfulness into mainstream medicine and society.

"Meditation does not involve trying to change your thinking by thinking some more. It involves watching thought itself. Another way to look at meditation is to view the process of thinking itself as a waterfall, a continual cascading of thought. In cultivating mindfulness, we are going beyond or behind our thinking, much the way you might find a vantage point in a cave or depression in the rock behind a waterfall. We still see and hear the water, but we are out of the torrent."

CHAPTER 36:

Other useful tools

Just as people have realized exercise is a must for their health and wellbeing in this technological age, I believe in the near future we'll realize the same is true for meditation and mindfulness. There is a lot of stuff we can do to decrease stress and mental overstimulation. Just like the explosion of gyms in developed countries, I think there will be an explosion of centers that teach and practice meditation and mindfulness.

Now that I'm through gazing into my magic crystal ball, let me share some of the other best mindfulness tools I've found.

Focused Breathing

This can range from the simple to the complex—from no more than taking 5-6 breaths with a higher level of attention, to yogic breathing exercises that fit under the umbrella of *pranayama* (a Sanskrit word meaning 'drawing out the life force'). If you want to go more deeply, I suggest you find a good yoga instructor and work with them directly.

For those who just want to try it out, here's a simple focused breathing exercise:

1. Sit comfortably.

2. Close your eyes.

3. Focus on your breath coming into and out of your body.

4. Breathe in deeply to the count of 4.

5. Breathe out deeply to the count of 6.

6. Repeat 5-10 times (or as long as you feel you want to).

Focused breathing is called 'healing breath' for a reason. It deactivates the stress response, utilizes the diaphragm, relaxes the stomach, draws more oxygen into the lungs, helps relax the body and muscles, and stimulates the activation of the relaxation response. It helps the body to heal by creating an environment that's conducive to self-healing.

As you breathe, aim to breathe into the stomach first (by relaxing the stomach muscles and using the diaphragm), then let the ribs expand and finally let your shoulders rise. The deepest breath does not come from lifting the shoulders up in the air. That's called tension! Our deepest breath comes by relaxing into the belly regions.

Velcro and Teflon

In his book *Hardwiring Happiness,* Rick Hanson makes a great statement. He says we're like Velcro for the bad and Teflon for the good. In other words, we readily notice and are attracted to the 'bad' and tend to not let in, or quickly move past, the 'good.' It's no one's fault. It's just part of our crazy evolution and in-built survival mechanisms. Back in the day (a few 100,000 years ago), we could only survive if we were hypersensitive to threats. So we got REALLY good at noticing all the things that could potentially go wrong. And that fixation on the 'bad' for all those millions of years means we're now subconsciously programmed to notice the bad and brush over the good.

All is not lost though. Hanson says we can do something about it—something he calls 'hardwiring happiness.'

How many times have you noticed something wrong and become fixated on it, playing around with it in your mind about a bazillion times? I don't know about you, but my hands up in the air. Compare that to the times you saw something nice or somebody said something nice to you and you kept on walking or went back to your business and forgot about it.

From a brain perspective, this lopsided focus is responsible for what we neurologically become and thus emotionally experience. So, time to make a change. Time for happiness — a state where positive thoughts exceed negative thoughts something like five to one. Time to change the odds in our favor!

Hardwiring Happiness

To hardwire more of the good we need to turn up the good by using a little psychology strategy we talked about earlier called the 'IF-THEN' strategy. If X happens then I do Y. It requires no additional thinking power at the time, as you have predetermined and thus preprogrammed your response.

Here's how to use this strategy to increase your happiness quotient. If you see, hear, feel, taste or touch something that makes you think, "That's nice" (or beautiful, interesting, amazing, etc.) THEN do the following:

1. Pause.

2. Bring your attention to it.

3. Deepen your attention of it.

4. Feel the goodness of it seeping through your body as you experience whatever it is.

5. Consciously deepen and expand those positive feelings.

This whole process only takes 15-30 seconds – so no excuses! However, it actually causes you, by directing your attention and engaging your feelings, to write a memory into your brain. The deeper the positive emotions the stronger the memory will be. This is also similar to gratitude exercises but more focused.

If you do this daily, several times a day, you'll actually rewire your brain towards the positive. You'll also be able to pull up these positive emotionally charged memories to reduce the emotional intensity of any bad experiences.

Examples:
- Seeing and hearing the ocean
- Looking up at a clear blue sky
- Finding a beautiful pebble or shell on the beach
- Looking at a beautiful tree
- Feeling sunshine on your face
- Seeing birds flying past
- Looking at a small flying insect

There are thousands of things each day that are amazing and usually go unnoticed. Life is not about getting excited about the big things. A beautiful life is about appreciating the small and regularly occurring things in life.

The resonance of your heart

The heart actually has its own independent nervous system with a plexus of about 40,000 nerve cells that act like a brain, which suggests a certain level of intelligence in the heart itself. Rollin McCraty explains in *The Energetic Heart*, "The heart generates the largest electromagnetic field in the body. The electrical field as measured in an electrocardiogram (ECG) is about 60 times greater in amplitude than the brain waves recorded in an electroencephalogram (EEG)."

Researchers at the Institute of HeartMath have been studying the heart to determine ways to help people reduce stress, self-regulate emotions, build energy and resilience and understand the impact of the heart on their health and well-being.

It's been observed that when subjects focus their attention on their hearts and then deliberately generate a core heart feeling such as love, appreciation or care, it causes their heart rhythms to become more coherent. This actually is a neural and biochemical response, which reduces the stress response and activates the relaxation response.

Something called Entrainment

Entrainment is cool and has nothing to do with trains. A good example of the principle of entrainment is when a number of grandfather clocks (the mechanical ones with a pendulum) are ticking away in a room together. The biggest of the clocks with the biggest pendulum somehow causes the other clocks to start ticking in its rhythm. It entrains (or influences) the other clocks.

The HeartMath Institute's studies show that the heart is the strongest biological oscillator in the human body. In fact, it's so strong it can pull the rest of the body's systems into entrainment with it. Which means when a person is in a loving or compassionate state, their heart's electromagnetic field is so strong it not only entrains and uplifts their own system, it can even entrain another's person's brain if they're standing within six feet!

So, mindfulness practice is not just about trying to still the monkey chatter in the mind (which can be frikkin hard), it's also HUGELY about directing your attention to your heart.

Focus on expanding the core heart feelings like love, compassion, caring and harmony. Feel the emotion spread through your whole body. That is your heart's harmony (and its powerful electromagnetic field) entraining your brain and every other part of your body to its rhythms.

The steps look like this:

1. Notice the mind going bonkers.

2. Bring your attention to your heart.

3. Imagine you're breathing into your heart with each inward breath and that with each outward breath your heart is relaxing and harmonizing.

4. Imagine love, compassion and peace building up in your heart. Feel it.

5. Just sit with that feeling in your heart and notice how it stills your racing mind.

6. Place your hand on your heart while you're feeling this strong positive emotion. This creates a neurological association between the act of placing your hand over your heart with the feeling in your heart so that in the future you can simply place your hand over your heart to generate and experience those same feelings. This is an NLP technique called 'anchoring.'

Breath Walking

I was first introduced to breath walking while listening to a Tony Robbins audio program. The concept is very simple and designed to still the thinking mind by paying so much attention to what you're physically doing that you have no residual capacity to form thoughts. It's another great way to calm down!

The basic method is:

1. Take four steps forward inhaling through your nose (without exhaling) as each foot touches the ground.

2. The next four steps forward you breathe OUT (without inhaling) as each foot touches the ground (breathing out the mouth is easier for beginners).

3. Then repeat the cycle. Four steps, four breaths' IN. Four steps, four breaths' OUT.

4. Pay particular attention to your foot placement, your breathing, your stride, your rhythm and you will have limited space left for random thoughts.

To see a demonstration of breath walking do a search on YouTube for 'carl massy breath walking.' I also mention in the video another layer you can add to the exercise to further still your mind if it continues to wander.

CHAPTER 37:

Pillar 5 (Mindfulness) Summary

When it comes to Mindfulness, this is what you need to know:

1. Our thoughts directly affect our health. When we're relaxed and not in a stress response, we're able to make better choices. We think more clearly, see more opportunities and are generally more creative.

2. When we have thoughts that cause a stress response and its accompanying toxic neurochemical cocktail, it adversely affects our cells' environment in the body. A chronic stress response will lead to significant health issues.

3. Deactivating the stress response is one of the keys to optimum health.

4. Much of the meaning we give things—both positive and negative—was programmed into us at an early age before we knew better and is below the threshold of our normal conscious attention.

5. We are only conscious of our thoughts, feelings and habitual behavior about five percent of the time. Most of the time we're on autopilot, which is great when the program is up-to-date and appropriate for the current conditions. But usually we're running on outdated and disempowering programs and habitual patterns. We need to update our thinking and beliefs as we go through life.

6. To do this we need to be conscious of our thoughts, beliefs, emotional patterns, and habitual behaviors so we have the option of choosing new thoughts, emotions and habits. This is not easy and requires diligence, but it can be done.

7. One way to do this is to slow down and become more conscious. We need

to tap into all of our senses. This gives us a better perspective, greater knowledge and enhanced wisdom so we're sufficiently informed to make the choices that attain better results.

8. Meditation is a great health tool in the over-stimulated world that we live in. It deactivates the stress response, reduces heart rate and blood pressure, and decreases muscle tension and oxygen consumption. Meditation is an incredible tonic for the mind and body.

9. There are many other mindfulness tools for reducing stress.

Optimum Health Strategies

1. Start meditating. Around 15-20 a day is highly effective for reducing stress and increasing healing. If that seems like a lot of time, start with 2 minutes a day and build up to 15 minutes a day.

2. Pay more attention to your thoughts. When you feel stressed, notice! What you are telling yourself to make you feel this way? Challenge the thought. Is the thought true 100 percent of the time in 100 percent of cases? If it is not, then it is not a FACT. So let it go. Find a more empowering belief.

3. Pay attention to the language you use when you speak to others. Is it empowering or disempowering? Is it motivating or critical? Are you exaggerating or sticking with reality? Become super conscious of your language today and for the rest of this week and know it affects your internal health.

4. Finish these sentences with at least 10-20 responses (the more responses you write, the deeper you are getting into uncovering your subconscious beliefs):
    *   When I slow down it makes me feel...
    *   When I slow down I think it will...

5. This exercise will help you determine what your beliefs are in relation to 'slowing down.' Perhaps you have beliefs that tell you unless you are superhuman and doing 20 things at once, you are not worthy or good enough or...?

Recommended Resources

There are a number of different sites with resources to help create a meditation practice. Some of them include:

- www.blissitations.com *(by the Entheos Academy)*
- www.centerpointe.com *(by Centerpointe Research Institute)*
- The Chopra Center
- UCLA Mindful Awareness Research Center
- The Institute of HeartMath

Try different Phone Apps like: The Mindfulness App, Meditate, Mindfulness Meditation, Breathe2Relax, Simply Being (I have not used these apps myself, but have listed them here to give you a start point).

Check out my iTunes Channel called *The Happiness Class* for an interview I did with meditation teacher Angela Perez on *'How to Meditate'*. It is another great resource to get you started and focused on people new to regular meditation.

Books:

- *You Are The Placebo* by Dr Joe Dispenza
- *Wherever You Go, There You Are* by Jon Kabat Zin
- *The Art of Meditation* by Matthieu Ricard
- *The Fire Starter* by Danielle LaPorte
- *Your Brain At Work* by David Rock
- *Evolve Your Brain* by Dr. Joe Dispenza
- *Breaking the Habit of Being Yourself* by Dr. Joe Dispenza
- *The Brain That Changes Itself* by Dr. Norman Doidge
- *Hardwiring Happiness* by Rick Hanson
- *Brain Rules* by John Medina
- *Brain Power* by Michael Gelb and Kelly Howell
- *Mind Over Medicine* by Lissa Rankin, MD

- *Overcoming Destructive Beliefs, Feelings and Behaviors* by Dr. Albert Ellis
- *The Tools* by Phil Stutz and Barry Michels

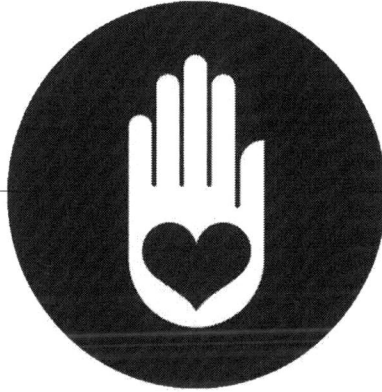

PILLAR 6
WHOLEHEARTEDNESS

*If you think dealing with issues like worthiness and authenticity
and vulnerability are not worthwhile because there are more pressing issues,
like the bottom line or attendance or standardized test scores,
you are sadly, sadly mistaken.
It underpins everything.*
Brene Brown, American research professor, author and speaker

CHAPTER 38:

What does the heart say?

The heart is so much more than just a pump and part of the circulatory system. The heart matters enormously, especially when it comes to attaining and maintaining optimum health because everything we involve ourselves in—our intimate relationships, our work and friendships—affects us at the level of the heart. If we're not following our hearts' desires and callings we're not doing our health any favors.

Happiness is more than the *absence* of negative emotions such as fear, worry, anger, rage, frustration, and disconnection. Happiness is the non-judgmental *inclusion* of all these states as part of our human experience and an expansion to include other feelings such as joy, fulfillment, anticipation, excitement, and love. A lot of New Age philosophy seems to reject uncomfortable emotions as 'negative.' But if someone tells you they never feel negative emotions you might wonder whether they feel anything at all.

I once coached a client in France and she talked about feeling nothing emotionally and that she was in a place devoid of enjoyment and meaning. Which is what happens when you remove heartfelt emotions, whether joy or sorrow, laughter or tears, fulfillment or rejection from life's equation. Without the vulnerability to feel everything, life ceases to have any meaning.

Emotions and the real you

Our emotions add color and vibrancy to life. Dr. Darren Weissman, author of

The Heart of the Matter, says that emotions are actually the *energy of creation in motion at a subtle level.* Just like the importance of blood flowing through the body, without the flow of emotional energy through our brain and body with its cocktail of chemicals and neurotransmitters stimulating everything, we're likely to lose touch with our feeling nature and suffer health issues as result.

Stop and think for a minute about who is more likely to achieve their goal? The person who has a great intellectual idea for getting to their goal, or the person who desires a goal with all their heart? Hands down it's the person whose heart and emotions are fully invested in their dream. Who is more likely to achieve success in a job or in a work relationship? A woman or man who is muddling along, feeling like they're just a cog in a wheel, or someone who feels like they're a valuable part of a team, adding to the work environment?

The latter of course.

Enthusiasm, inspiration, passion, excitement, and, of course, love, are the biggie emotions we associate with the heart. All these emotions are tremendously powerful and motivating. Experiencing them shows us that we're operating with openness and vulnerability. Why? Because it's not possible to be passionate and not vulnerable. When you're passionate about something your whole heart and soul are in it. You're 'out there' for the whole world to see. Yes, this kind of vulnerability can lead to pain and suffering. But that's just part of the package called life. Despite what we're taught to think, it's ALL good. Vulnerability means we're not dragging around a boatload of heavy armor and defensive issues, trying to protect ourselves from threats, both real and imagined.

Brené Brown, author of *Daring Greatly*, defines wholeheartedness as:

"The capacity to engage in our lives with authenticity, cultivate courage and compassion, and embrace — not in that self-help-book, motivational-seminar way, but really, deeply, profoundly embrace—the imperfections of who we really are."

Yes, we're all imperfect. (Even me!) And it's incredibly easy to get defensive about our weaknesses and uncertainties. We want to be looking good all the time to all the people around us. Right? But this just isn't realistic—it isn't being real.

The thing is, when your heart's engaged you're being the most authentic you possible. You aren't worried about how your hair looks (well, maybe you are and that's okay) but what I mean is, you're not stiff and hung-up about everything. You're too busy doing what you love to be overly concerned about what others think. You're too busy being authentic. And when you're being authentic not only are you jazzed emotionally, you're in alignment with your greatest truth: the truth of who you really are.

When you're wholehearted, the outside environment matches the inside you. One reflects the other. And that means you're in the flow. Everything is lined up and in harmony—mind, body, spirit, and action. This doesn't mean everything automatically goes perfectly in life (dang!). Life is life after all and stuff happens. But when you're doing what you love you've got a greater ability to handle the crap when it does show up.

Emotions and illness

There are many things impacting our health which are often overlooked by the existing medical system—aspects of our lives that we don't often associate with our health, which, on closer inspection, are major causes of everything from stomach problems, to headaches, to back pain, to cancer, to diabetes, shoulder pain, eye problems, hearing difficulties, indigestion—you name it.

Dr. Weissman (who I like to call Dr. D) says flat out *"Without exception, subconscious emotions are the source of all disease."*

Wow. How is that possible?

As I said before, the time emotions stop being okay for our health and happiness is when we (and they) get STUCK (kind of like a blood clot). Just like the circulatory system, if our emotions get stuck in our body or suppressed because we don't want to deal with them, they cause physical symptoms to show up. And a LOT of emotions get suppressed.

Ever experience your parents yelling at you, telling you, "Don't get angry at your sister! Don't pout! Stop feeling sorry for yourself!" Where do these emotions we're not supposed to be feeling and expressing go? They go straight into our subconscious and just sit there, waiting to be expressed so they can MOVE on.

And then there's emotional trauma—things that happen to us that are so terrible we just can't emotionally handle it at the time—like child molestation, rape or a severe accident or war.

Stuffing away emotions we're told we shouldn't feel or are unequipped to handle at the time of a trauma is a brilliant survival mechanism of the mind. But the 30-year-old you isn't the same as the 6-year-old you. Once we grow up, we need to feel the painful, upsetting emotions we had to lock away and process them to learn and grow and let their stuck energies naturally dissipate.

As Dr. D puts it: "For optimal health and wellbeing, longevity and purposeful life expression, humans must learn how emotions function in their lives and learn how to effectively process the emotions they experience as they happen. We also must learn how to access emotions that, through youth and inexperience and inability, we have stuffed away in our subconscious. Once there, if unattended, they wreak all sorts of havoc!"

They sure do. And what's really interesting is that there's a direct correlation between our emotional wounds and the kinds of problems and symptoms that these unexpressed emotions trigger in the body.

Louise Hay is one of the founders of the self-help movement, and her first book, *Heal Your Body*, was published in 1976. It ended up selling millions of copies and was translated into 25 languages. In it, she discusses the connection between mind, emotions, life circumstances and the body's health, citing case after case where emotional problems in jobs, relationships, and the home environment show up as specific health problems with the body. For example, she discovered that lower back pain is often emotionally related to problematic financial issues or feeling unsupported in life.

Just this morning I got out of bed feeling lower back pain (which I've had for days) and realized I needed to dig into it deeply to discover what the root cause was. As I focused deep into the pain in my back I realized that, although my finances were cool, there was an emotional block I was experiencing in a business relationship I was involved in. I realized I felt completely unsupported by the other party. Once I processed the issue of feeling unsupported (a process I'll get into in the next chapter) and could look at the situation from a perspective of knowledge and compassion, I was then able to wisely decide the course of action I needed to take.

And guess what? When I got out of my 'stuckness' and let all that emotional energy flow through me, 'miraculously' my lower back pain subsided.

Remember, we're holistic beings. Our mind, body and emotions are all linked. And how else can we know when something's wrong except to either know it mentally, or feel it through our body? Either way our body is the key to the whole thing—*it's the vehicle through which life circumstances communicate*. And it's fascinating how appropriately the body mirrors the message.

If you have an inflexible body, you're likely to have an inflexible mind and vice versa. If you have trouble expressing yourself or voicing your truth, you might manifest a physical inability to speak up, or have issues with the throat, like hypothyroidism, or a goiter. Hip aches and pains tend to reflect that you are out of balance emotionally or in how you are living your life.

If we're living halfheartedly, settling for intimate relationships that are less than satisfactory, careers we don't like, and dealing with work relationships that are stressful or downright mean-spirited, after awhile we can definitely expect problems in the heart area to show up—from acid reflux to heart palpitations to a heart attack or heart failure.

I don't mean to scare you—but then maybe I do if that's what it takes for you to start realizing how much impact emotional difficulties have on your health. It took this ex-army boy a long time to make his way to understanding the heart and emotions and how vital they are. I can assure you, if you are all in your head and limited as far as heart expression is concerned, you'll miss out on most of the richness this life has to offer.

CHAPTER 39:

The Heart of the Matter

One of my favorite teachers, people and authors is Dr. Darren Weissman. He developed the *LifeLine Technique®*, an extremely powerful mind-body modality for processing emotions. He is also the author of a book I highly recommend, called *The Heart of the Matter*, co-authored with my fantastic editor, Cate Montana. I liked the book title so much I co-opted it for the title of this chapter (also known as pinching it)!

I cannot stress enough the importance of getting right with your emotions. You can jog until you drop, have the tightest abs, eat right, do yoga—and if you're emotionally shut-down or running a bunch of negative emotional programs none of it's worth a damn because if you feel like crap on the inside, what good does the rest do?

Over and over I've tried to impress upon you that the mind and body and emotions and spirit are not separate things. You are a symphony in motion and if the whole symphony is playing great together but the lead violin is out of key, whacking away on another tune altogether, the whole thing sounds (and feels) terrible.

Aligning mind and emotions

Your heart is the lead violin in your orchestra.

Remember, the heart generates the largest electromagnetic field in the body.

It can entrain your brain. It can entrain other people's brains. It has its own plexus of nerves that serves as a 'mini-brain' and the heart actually can hijack the brain altogether and take it for a ride. How many times have you had the experience of simply responding to a situation, helping somebody or doing something for someone before you could even think about it? That's your heart in action.

Unfortunately we live in a world where the mind is given greater credibility and importance than the heart. We're taught to be logical and ruthless, to suppress our emotions and look out for #1. (And look where that's got us.)

We have thousands of thoughts that enter our mind every day. I think the official number is about 60,000 but I have no clue how scientists came up with it. Whether it's 60,000 or 54,763, the point is, we have lots of thoughts. The not so great thing is the vast majority are repetitive and negative — and we're taught to give even these blokes precedence over our feelings!

Most of these 60,000 thoughts come and go with minimal impact on us. But when we focus our conscious mind and attention on a particular thought, at that point we breathe life into it, giving it meaning and starting a biochemical response in our brain. The thought signals the release of neurotransmitters, neuropeptides and hormones into the blood stream and activates the autonomic nervous system. The thought now has a corresponding physiological emotional response to it, and, depending on the thought, it's created either a Bloody Mary or a Green Smoothie for you to digest.

This is how the thought/emotion process generally flows:

1. Thoughts come to mind.

2. You give attention to a thought.

3. You give meaning to that thought.

4. The relevant electrical and biochemical response is activated based on the

meaning triggering emotions.

5.   The body responds chemically and your emotions run wild.

If the emotional/chemical response is strong enough, a feedback loop can occur.

Let's say your boss just gave somebody else the promotion you've been promised. You're angry and hurt and your thoughts create angry, wounded emotions. You feel terrible. You feel betrayed. You feel insignificant. These chemical emotional reactions to your thoughts called e-motions in turn create more thoughts that resonate to the frequency of anger and woundedness. These thoughts in turn trigger more corresponding emotions, which in turn create more hurt thoughts, until you're in a total fury.

This is what's commonly called 'having a meltdown.'

From the last section on Mindfulness we know it's definitely possible (but not necessarily easy) to control this process by CHOOSING where to place your attention via your powerful conscious mind, and deciding what meaning you give to a thought. We can change the meaning of a situation and our corresponding thoughts about it from thoughts of anger to thoughts of neutrality, or even thoughts of positivity and growth.

Instead of over-reacting and slamming our boss, we can choose calmness and go have an adult talk and find out what happened. Maybe our emotional volatility is what made her or him pass us over for that promotion in the first place. Thing is, unless we consciously choose to modulate our thoughts and emotions, we'll never be in a place where we can find out and get the important information we need to understand the situation so we can CHANGE. We'll just storm around feeling angry and hurt until we either quit or get fired or fall over sick.

The meaning we give things determines how we feel, and it is our feelings that truly define our life. So, before we leave the promotion fiasco, I want to show you how being highly sensitive and aware of subtle feelings/emotions can take you down a whole different path. Ready?

You find out you haven't gotten the promotion.

Remember the point about SLOWING DOWN and how important that is? If you're practicing mindfulness there's the possibility that when you get the news you'll be SLOWED-DOWN enough and in touch with yourself enough that you'll notice what's really going on in your psyche when you get the news.

Perhaps the news initially triggers a fleeting sense of relief. This is a message to you: *I didn't really want that promotion. It would have caused too much stress, taken me away from the kids... I don't really even like what I do...* This is a whole different meaning/thought/emotion track than anger and hurt—a meaning track that just may lead you to finding another job or even a new career.

Perhaps the news initially triggers a sense of guilt and the words in your head that accompany that guilt are: *I'm not good enough. I'm a loser. I can't do anything right.* You've just been mindful enough to catch a subtle underlying core belief about yourself that needs conscious addressing. No wonder you got passed over for a promotion! This glimpse into yourself opens up a whole new meaning track where you get the opportunity to start working on some inner false beliefs about yourself, which takes you down the road of self-empowerment and maybe even the next promotion.

Look what you miss by being 'unconscious' and unreflective and un-self-aware. Look what you miss when your mind and emotions are on autopilot!

To change the meaning of something we need to be open to seeing it from another perspective. Instead of automatically thinking the worst (my boss is a jerk; I've been screwed) we need to ask ourselves 'what else could this mean?'

For instance, when we get a confusing text message from our partner, instead of making an assumption that causes a stress response, we ask ourselves "what else could it mean?" Maybe it's that damn spell check thing, or they were in a rush, or they assumed you would understand, or they sent the message to the wrong person. A different meaning causes a different emotional/physical response, which leads to healing or to stress.

Handling suppressed emotions

I don't want to give the impression that there's something wrong with being angry or hurt. These are natural reactions to being disappointed. Maybe your boss really is a jerk. Maybe the whole thing really was unfair. And even if it wasn't unfair you still have the right to feel like you really feel and think what you think.

Healthy balanced emotions and thoughts are not about suppressing stuff. It's about being appropriate and conscious of what you're doing. If you need to rant for a while, then rant! Get it on and get it over with. Expressing emotions is better than suppressing them. Just don't get carried away and let your thoughts and emotions flush you down the drain.

Unfortunately, we've all been taught since infancy to suppress and disguise our emotions. As a result, we all have suppressed emotions locked away in our subconscious that are affecting our health and happiness.

As Dr. Darren points out in *The Heart of the Matter*: "Every thought we think bears an emotional charge that can alter body chemistry and heart and brain rhythms. Depending upon the frequency signature of the e-motion, emotional effects can range from highly positive and transformative to highly destructive. If unresolved, suppressed, and left misunderstood, emotions can wreak all sorts of havoc, forming the roots of suffering."

If we want to experience optimum health and happiness in our lives, we need to 1) be mindful enough to get in touch with our real emotions and then 2) come up with ways to process them.

One of the ways Dr. D teaches people to process emotions (which is covered in full detail in *The Heart of the Matter*), is called the *See, Feel, Hear Technique*. I will cover a part of it briefly here—enough so you will realize the strength and brilliant simplicity of it.

Essentially, when you first become aware of a negative emotion, SLOW DOWN. Consciously observe it. Then you close your eyes and from the perspective of an observer, tune into the emotion. Consciously ask to SEE any images associated with the emotion. Watch them as they come up when you connect to that emotion. For example, let's say you've gotten in touch with the emotion of feeling insignificant—an emotion you felt when you missed that promotion.

Don't judge or get involved, just watch what comes up. Maybe it's a scene in your front yard when you were four and your dad was tossing you a ball and you couldn't catch it with your little chubby hands. There is no right or wrong. Just see the images. Say "thank you" to the images with compassion and gratitude once you've finished watching.

Next, consciously FEEL the emotions those images trigger in your body. Perhaps you feel guilt. Where do you feel it? What does it feel like? Really get into the feeling. Then again, say "thank you" with compassion and gratitude. Finally get in touch with what the feeling has to say. What do you HEAR? What is the inner voice and internal dialogue saying when you connect with this emotion? Maybe you hear kids on a playground taunting you, crying "loser!" Maybe it's your dad telling you not to be so "clumsy."

Just listen without judgment. Observe. Say "thank you" with gratitude, compassion, and love. Now, is there more?

Did the voices in your head trigger another emotion? Did the word "loser" make you feel something else? Maybe instead of guilt, you now feel anxiety. Go through the whole SEE, FEEL, HEAR process again, this time processing the emotion of anxiety. What images arise? What voices? Keep cycling through the SEE, FEEL, HEAR process until no more negative associations come up to consciousness.

Now, take a moment to imagine how you would like to be.

Instead of feeling insignificant (your starter emotion) perhaps you'd like to feel valuable. Go through the SEE, FEEL, HEAR process again, this time starting with seeing images of being valuable, feeling valuable and hearing what 'valuable' has to say.

This technique, when done fully, is about learning and processing and letting go of the stories that hold negative emotions in place in the subconscious, then replacing them with more healthy emotions. It may seem simple (and it is), but it's incredibly powerful. Why? Because this is what your subconscious wants you to do: Evolve! Grow! Move on!

To learn the whole technique, check out Dr. D's book.

Getting to the place where you know that, "Even though I was feeling this, I am okay. I accept who I am," is a powerful place. It's the antidote to fear and self-judgment. It's also about connecting with your heart and emotions and realizing their powerful role in your health.

When your heart is lit up with love and compassion for yourself and others, it contributes to the health of your body and the wellbeing of the whole rest of the world.

CHAPTER 40:

Tips for increasing wholeheartedness

What inspires whole-heartedness?

When I lived in Greece and Italy I paid particular attention to how the people there lived. They ate pasta, drenched everything in olive oil and drank red wine. They sat up drinking coffee until the wee hours. They napped during the day.

Few of these things seem 'healthy' to the Western mind, even though now scientists say red wine is good for you because of antioxidants called polyphenols (in particular resveratrol). As you know, I don't consider alcohol to be a health food. It's acidic in nature when our body is more likely to thrive on an alkaline diet, and too much alcohol has adverse effects on the liver. As far as I'm concerned, if you want the antioxidant effects of red wine, eat a handful of red grapes, which have even more antioxidants, fiber, and phytonutrients.

But I'm missing my own point here, which is that I don't think it's so much the alcohol contributing to the good health of people living in the Mediterranean as it is the benefits and interpersonal relationships that occur while sharing a glass of red wine. When families come together to share food and wine, they also share another extremely healing substance called 'each other.' For me, it's not the wine but the environment created around wine that is health-giving. It's the caring and laughter, the compassion, love and supportive ears... the connection. All these things are healing for the body because they deactivate the STRESS response and activate the RELAXATION response.

In *The Honeymoon Effect,* by Dr. Bruce Lipton, he asks people to think back to a time when they fell in love. And I'll ask you the same thing. How was your health at the time? Did you have more energy? Were you in great shape? Did you radiate vitality?

There are definitely healing benefits with this invisible thing called 'love,' and I highly encourage you to seek out ways to generate the feeling. As we've seen, you can consciously choose your emotions. You can process negative emotions and make room for the positive ones to grow. And you can set up your external environment to help bring more love and connections into your life as well.

How are your intimate relationships?

When you're in a healthy relationship you feel more supported and connected. You have a compassionate ear to listen to your problems and an extra person on the team to problem-solve. In a healthy relationship your stress levels are likely to be lower and activated for shorter periods of time. And when stress is not present the body is doing the self-healing thing.

What constitutes a positive and healthy intimate relationship? Well, here's my take on the subject. Healthy relationships include these things:

- Emotional and physical support

- Mutual respect for individual differences

- Positively encouraging

- No judgment

- Supportive of each others' individual goals and growth

- Equal energy put into the relationship

- Fidelity – both physical and emotional

- Physically intimate

- Playful

- High levels of integrity

- Ability to be authentically yourself

All of these things, with the exception of those points relating to sexual intimacy, should be qualities defining all the other relationships in your life. Whether it is friends and family or the greater community, bottom line, healthy relationships support a healthy body and mind.

Meaning-FULL Work

One of the main keys to happiness is the need to feel that our life is meaningful. Without a sense of meaning we're more likely to cling to immediate gratification and pleasures in order to feel good about things in the moment. We're also unlikely to have the desire and willpower to delay gratification and do the things we know to be necessary for optimum health. Without meaning it's even difficult to get out of bed in the morning because what's the point?

Since work constitutes a significant part of our life—whether it's paid work or work running a household and taking care of children—if what we do is *meaningless* to us we're unlikely to be happy and unlikely to take care of ourselves.

Frankly, I believe each one of us has skills, talents and dreams that are uniquely ours, aligned with the most authentic part of ourselves. You could even call it the divinely unique part of ourselves. Whether we're working as a baker, builder, consultant, waiter, miner, policewoman or dressmaker, when we're doing what feels like our souls' calling—when we've had the courage to follow that calling and live it each and every day, then we're being true to ourselves. And that's the foundation for happiness and good health.

If you have an inner calling but suppress it or pretend it's not there, it's like telling yourself you don't matter. And you will eventually experience health issues because of it. Doing work you hate is not only soul destroying, but (surprise!) it's bad for you physically. The knee issue you think is related to playing football in your teens might actually be related to feeling trapped in a job surrounded by people you don't respect. I've had clients with on-going physical ailments that suddenly cleared up when they changed jobs, or changed professions entirely and followed their calling.

You owe it to yourself (and life) to give what you want to do a shot. American mythologist and author Joseph Campbell would say, "Follow your bliss and don't be afraid, and doors will open where you didn't know they were going to be." In fact, Campbell would call this *'the hero's journey.'*

When you respond to your calling, you liberate a *power* within you that is much stronger than the *force* it takes to do something your heart isn't in. Bringing this back to optimum health, when you align yourself with your strengths and authentic calling, you liberate energy and increase your vitality. You change your vibrational energy and add to the overall health of your physical body, in particular that major organ called the heart.

The power of being in alignment with their inner calling is what gave Gandhi the ability to stand up to the British Empire. It's the same thing Susan Boyle drew on when she sang *I Dreamed a Dream* at her audition for Britain's Got Talent. It isn't a person's *force* that moves a billion people. It's the *power* unleashed when someone bares their authentic soul and operates from their heart.

When you *follow your bliss* you discover more about who you really are. You grow at a greater rate. And that job you're so afraid of leaving? Something like it will always be there. If worst came to worst I could go back to security consulting for the mega events tomorrow if I wanted to. But leaving that old job opened me up to a life I'd previously only dreamed of. Not because I'm able to buy super yachts now (I definitely cannot), but because I love what I do and I love the difference I make in peoples lives. The work I do is so aligned with my calling that sometimes even the obstacles feel like fun. And it's definitely made me tap into more of my potential.

So, what is your hearts desire? Are you ready to expose it to the light? To step into it? To give it a go? To step out of your comfort zone, pass through the discomfort zone, which is generally much smaller than we imagine, and arrive in the field of possibility? What would it take for you to give your dream the attention it is calling for and thoroughly deserves?

The 10-year question

When a particularly big life decision or opportunity that might simultaneously scare and excite you arises, ask yourself the question: "In ten years will I regret not having taken this opportunity (or life direction)?"

A heart-based answer will most likely give you a *feeling* of, "Hell yes I'll regret it!" This kind of gut-level, heart-level reaction means it's right to take on the challenge. If you're not 'feeling it' then maybe you're right to let it go.

The heart is a great resource and yardstick when it comes to getting the best out of life. When you want something 'with all your heart' you are very likely to achieve it. Conversely if your 'heart is not in it' whatever you're trying to do is likely to be a struggle. So listen to your heart. What is it telling you? Where do you need to be? With whom? What do you need to change? What do you need to let go of?

Remember, we all have a very powerful internal human need to grow physically, mentally, spiritually and emotionally. If we're not growing, we will deeply feel that something isn't right. This is true for relationships. jobs, dreams, health, you name it. Following your heart is definitely the way to optimum health, happiness and vitality.

An evolutionary need

One of our greatest desires is to feel intimacy. One of our greatest fears is to feel rejection. Sometimes we don't say 'hello' to someone as we walk past on a quiet section of the beach because we fear they may not say hello back. So instead of chancing rejection, we close off our hearts. We don't connect and thus we support the idea of separation.

There is a hypothesis that suggests we are terrified of rejection at a deep level because for thousands of years if we were banished from our tribe it would most likely mean our death. Acceptance means physical protection of the tribe and the feeling of security that goes with it. So we have subconsciously associated isolation, loneliness, disconnection and rejection with fear of death.

As a result, all these emotions are deeply stressful.

The person who feels they have no support and have to do everything themselves will constantly be on alert and in a stress response. Never mind the feelings are based on an inherited false belief. These feelings still have negative physical effects on our health.

I'm writing this on a flight coming back from Australia where I attended my 25-year (Class of '89) reunion graduating from the Royal Military College Duntroon. It might have been inconvenient and a challenge for a lot of us to get there, but the joy and (dare I say it?) love that was shared over those two days was life giving at the highest level. So take it from me and take the time and make the effort to support and maintain those quality relationships with friends and family in your life – they will add quality years to your life as well

CHAPTER 41:
Pillar 6 (Wholeheartedness) Summary

When it comes to Wholeheartedness, this is what you need to know:

1. You can be doing all of the best physical things for yourself with nutrition, physical activity, rest, detoxification and mindfulness, but if you are in a toxic relationship, in a job you hate, or feeling like life has no meaning, you are unlikely to be in optimum health. More likely you will be ill and have constant physical and mental health issues.

2. When we're guided by our hearts, we feel and know things that we cannot intellectually explain. The heart's promptings are messages from our deepest self telling us what's in our best interest. When our hearts are fully connected to the moment and we're listening to what our hearts say, we're stepping into the healing zone.

3. When we are in love, we are actually likely to be happiest and healthiest. Our health is positively or negatively affected by the quality of the relationships we have in our lives.

4. We need to process our emotions and keep them flowing to ensure we remain in the optimum health zone. Suppressing our emotions or getting 'stuck' in negative emotions affects our health and leads to physical and mental ailments.

5. Doing meaning-full work is important. If you're not doing work you find meaningful it will reduce your level of happiness and have a negative impact on your health.

Optimum Health Strategies

1. Wherever you are right now, be compassionate towards yourself. Say to yourself, "Even though I am feeling XYZ (or experiencing this symptom), I deeply and completely accept myself."

2. Do an audit of your life. Are you doing meaningful work? Are you in a quality relationship? (Does it need some work? Is it worth the work? Or do you need to move on?) Are you following your dreams?

3. Seek professional help—a counselor, a social worker, a life coach, a psychologist or therapist—to deal with emotional issues in your life that seem overwhelming. Find help that works for you.

4. Another great strategy for getting insight into your thinking and emotions is to write in a journal. Putting things down on paper can often add great clarity to a situation.

Recommended Resources

Check out some of Brene Brown's presentations on *YouTube*. Just do a search on: Brene Brown TED Talk Vulnerability. It is well worth watching.

Books:

*   *Daring Greatly* by Brene Brown
*   *The Fire Starter Sessions* by Danielle LaPorte
*   *The Heart of the Matter* by Dr. Darren Weissman and Cate Montana
*   *You Can Heal Your Life* by Louise Hay
*   *Loving What Is* by Byron Katie
*   *Tapping Solution* by Nick Ortner
*   *Mind Over Medicine* by Lissa Rankin

CHAPTER 42:

Facing Bad News

Preventative measures set us up for a high likelihood of optimum health. But these measures aren't a guarantee because the human being is a complex system and the bigger picture for our lives is mostly unknown. Our plan is to stack the odds heavily in our favor by following the guidelines in each of the 6 Pillars. But again, life brings surprises. So one of the last things I want to do is bring everything together in the context of having a serious illness.

What I would do if I got really bad news

Just to reiterate: I am not a doctor or a medical practitioner. I'm not offering a prescription for treating illness. I'm offering you insight into what I would do if I got really bad news. If you are facing severe health issues, I strongly encourage you to explore a treatment plan with the right range of professionals that seem appropriate to you. But, at the same time, do consider ALL 6 Pillars.

Now, let's look at what Carl Massy would do if he was advised he had a serious disease.

Firstly, I would see this disease as an opportunity to learn. It is what it is, right now; so how can I grow from this experience?

I know I'm getting a vital message from my subconscious mind via my body, telling me something is not right, that some BIG action needs to be taken in my life. I also know it means my conscious awareness of everything — my body's needs, my emotional needs, my home and work situations — must step up to a whole new level. I'd look for mental, emotional and physical things that may be causing an imbalance in my body. At the same time I would take the following specific actions:

1. I would continue doing physical activity, but I would probably increase activities like yoga and Qigong that go beyond a purely physical workout. Plus add in more fun stuff like freestyle dancing.

2. I would aim for 9-10 hours sleep a night. I would also take regular breaks through the day, working for 45 minutes and then breaking for 15 minutes. I would reduce my work week down to 4 days and make sure that at least 1-2 days were completely technology free. I would also take a 3-5 day time-out every month.

3. I would follow a 100 percent whole-food, plant-based diet. I would remove 100 percent of processed food from my diet. I would increase the amount of juicing in a day to load up on even more micronutrients. I would aim for 100 percent organic. I would also get a great water filter.

4. I would slow down and become more conscious of my eating. I would aim to increase the amount of times I chewed my food. The aim of my eating would be nourishment, connection to the food, plus appreciation.

5. I would do a MAJOR detoxification of my body under the supervision of a professional team. Most likely I'd take a retreat with a holistic focus on mind, body and spirit. I would search for any toxins (physical and/or emotional) and remove them from my life, replacing physical things with natural alternatives.

6. I would have two massages each week to help lymph flow and the removal of toxins.

7. I would increase my meditation practice to 1 hour each day (I currently meditate 15-30 minutes daily).

8. I would remind myself often to slow down and smell the roses. I would spend more time in nature, walking and meditating.

9. I would do more journaling and writing. Every day I would write down 10 things I am grateful for (currently this is a verbal daily practice for me).

10. I would practice generating feelings of love and gratitude frequently throughout the day. I would act with even more compassion towards others and ESPECIALLY towards myself. I would say one of Louise Hay's favorite mantras, "I love and approve of myself," at least a 100 times a day. I would say thank you even more than I do now.

11. I would stop watching movies with any violence in them (I do love action movies) and watch feel-good movies only—stuff like The Blind Side or Invictus or old song and dance movies with greats like Fred Astaire, Ginger Rodgers and Gene Kelly. I'd watch feel-good romantic comedies (Yes, chick-flicks!)

12. I'd get the advice of an integrative medical practitioner who is trained in both western medicine and alternative therapies that practices detoxing, nutrition and other health modalities. I'm not adverse to the medical profession. I'm just adverse to the pharmaceutical industry and impersonal pill-popping solutions to optimum health.

13. I would do the emotional and mental work to ensure there are no unprocessed emotional issues affecting the healing of my body and keeping it in a stress response. This might include hypnotherapy, Emotional Freedom Technique (Tapping), Neuro Linguistic Programming, Timeline Therapy®, The LifeLine Technique®, Reiki, kinesiology, psychotherapy, and any other methods that I come across along the way. One of my preferred healing methods, as I write this book, is The LifeLine Technique® by Dr. Darren Weissman. It is thorough, deep and not dependent on the conscious mind 'doing' anything.

14. I would step back and perform a complete audit of my work. I would focus more on the stuff I love and that makes a difference to other people.

I would stop doing stuff that doesn't matter. I would connect more fully with my passion and purpose in life. I would ensure that my work fulfilled me and was a physical expression of love flowing to and through me. I would also look at removing or reducing any stressors that existed in my work.

15. I would spend more time with the people that I love and NO time at all with people who suck on my energy, whine, complain and generally make me feel worse. I would look at how I could improve my intimate relationship even more, taking it to an even deeper level. I would make sure I wasn't holding back love or carrying around any resentment or frustration. I would put more love into all of the relationships in my life.

16. I would look for stuff that was 'undone.' Is there an experience I've been putting off? A burning desire to do something? A place I want to visit? I can't think of too many things. I've lived a very full life packed with amazing experiences because I've always chosen to spend my money on experiences instead of physical possessions (at this point I haven't owned a car since the year 2000).

17. Finally, I would look at how I could give a little more. What charity things could I do and get involved in? Is there a need I could contribute to? Where could I best use my talents, time and energy in the service of others?

It's an interesting exercise figuring out what I'd do. What would your list look like?

As I wrote these 17 points down, the question popped into my head: "Why aren't you doing all these things now?" Hmmm. I'm doing most. But most isn't all. Now is the time for me to truly own that list and see where I could improve my life even more, NOW, TODAY, before I get sick.

Here are the areas I know I can improve on:
1.   Eat less processed food. I eat very little. But I do have a sweet tooth that

runs the show sometimes, especially when I'm travelling for work.

2. I need to take one work-free, technology-free day a week. I need to take more breaks through the day rather than working like a 17th century coal miner.

3. I will cut down on the kill 'em, gruesome action movies and replace them with nicer movies.

4. I will make an effort to spend more time with people I admire who leave me feeling great afterwards.

5. I will review my work and work-related activities to minimize the high stress, low value things I still do.

6. I will do more charity work.

CHAPTER 43:

Summary

The following is a brief summary of what measures to take if you want optimum health in your life:

1. Be physically active most days of the week. Mix the activities up so you are getting a mix of aerobic, resistance, stretching, active mind-body, and play.

2. Get adequate rest each night. Aim for 7.5 to 9 hours sleep a night.

3. Take mini breaks throughout the day. Have at least one day off a week where you do no work and preferably disconnect from technology like cell phones, tablets and computers. Take an annual vacation and regular mini breaks throughout the year.

4. Eat food as close to nature as possible. Significantly reduce the amount of processed food in your diet. Remove as much sugar (all kinds) from your diet as possible. Reduce the amount of animal-based food in your diet. Don't drink flavored drinks, which are loaded with sugar. Also go easy on dairy and gluten from highly processed grain products.

5. Cleanse your body on a regular basis. Aim for one time per year where you do a major detox. Drink a daily Green Drink for a micronutrient overload and body cleanse. Reduce the amount of non-naturally occurring chemicals around the household.

6. Drink more pure water.

7. Practice meditation. Slow down as you move through your day, so you can be more conscious of the decisions you make. Pay attention to your thinking and the words you use. Pay attention to your behaviors to ensure they are responsive and not reactive. Pay attention to your breath, and keep

it long and deep.

8. When you become stressed, practice a mindfulness exercise to deactivate your stress response.

9. Surround yourself with people who allow and encourage you to be yourself. Spend time in high quality relationships.

10. Choose work that you love.

11. Get comfortable with saying 'no.'

12. Focus on having and buying experiences with nature and other people over owning material possessions.

TA DA! I just summarized this whole book in 12 bullet points!

I hope you haven't jumped to the end and think that this is all the information you need. We have to actively take the journey ourselves to discover the messages and meaning and experiences *behind* these brief words. We have to embrace and embody ALL the information to create optimum health.

CHAPTER 44:

In Conclusion

Take care of your body with steadfast fidelity.
The soul must see through these eyes alone, and if they are dim,
the whole world is clouded.
Johann Wolfgang von Goethe, German writer and statesman

Firstly, thank you for taking the time to read this book.

Time is one of the most precious commodities we have in life, so I don't take your commitment lightly. I also want to thank you for giving me a reason to spend the many hours tapping away with two fingers on my keyboard over this last year. Telling you what I've learned, researching more deeply into each topic, I've increased my own knowledge of the 6 Pillars to Optimum Health. Writing this book has also caused me to look at how I can make improvements in my own life.

A great quote from Jim Rohn, one of the great motivational speakers and authors of last century, comes to mind at this point:

What is easy to do is also easy not to do.

I'm sure much of what I've shared with you is knowledge you already had to some extent. But *knowing* is not enough. It's the *doing* that changes the outcome of your health. Just as Jim Rohn suggests, it's easy to do what you know is best for you. But it's also easy to let things slip until what was once a little thing, becomes a major illness or disease.

One of the major things I wanted to introduce into the optimum health equation is the role the mind and heart play in our physical health. An average fitness trainer who believes it's all about harder workouts and eating less carbs is missing an enormous part of what health is all about.

I also talked extensively about the need to activate the parasympathetic nervous system, better known as the *Relaxation Response*, to bring the body back into homeostasis, optimum health and harmony. We need to deeply understand the impact of stress on our bodies and become more conscious of the choices we're making and how they add to or lessen our stress levels. Some stress is okay and even necessary for growth. But consistent stress depletes the health of the cells in our bodies.

A high level of health, energy and vitality is needed to achieve the greatest results in life. When we have optimum health it's like we're poised on the starting blocks to a 100-meter race, ready to explode down the track towards the final destination. The track is your life's journey and the destination is one of your choosing. The greater vitality and energy you have, the greater the clarity of your mind, the higher level of your conscious awareness, the greater your life will be. So this book is not just about optimum health, it's about you being able to fully express the greatest version of your best and divine self.

Lastly, I want to say that you already have all you need within you, right now, to be an exceptional leader. You have the capacity to create the environment, both internally and externally that is most conducive to the optimum functioning of your body, mind, emotions, spirit and your life itself. You have the ability to lead your amazing mind and body to optimum health. You have the tools, the knowledge, the tips, the strategies and the support to be the best you can be.

I wish you the very best for your onwards and upwards journey in life. May you have an amazing time exploring and experiencing some amazing destinations along the way.

Remember, I'm here if you ever need me. I'll be that voice over your shoulder (or in your head) reminding you of what you know and of the potential that rests within you. Keep me posted on the challenges and wins on your journey and I look forward to sharing them. Maybe one day we'll step out of virtual space and meet in person. It'll be a lucky day for both of us if we do.

All the very best and take care.

Continuing Your Journey to Optimum Health

I am SO grateful you joined me on this healing journey and I look forward to serving you and crossing paths many times in the weeks, months and years to come.

If you want to fire some questions my way, or just reach out and say 'hi,' just drop into my **Carl Massy Facebook Page** and connect up. I would love to hear from you and love to hear what you learned reading this book.

You can also track me down and get some great free resources at **www.carlmassy.com**.

Also, I would be SO GRATEFUL (really I would), if you would do me the honor of leaving a comment on *Amazon* or *Goodreads* or the likes, to let me (and others know) what you thought of this book. It's through your support that I can continue to serve by taking my message that 'all of us are greatly in control of our health' to a broader audience.

If you want to continue your journey to optimum health and the best version of yourself possible, I would love to continue being your guide. I have a number of programs, workshops and retreats that have been of great benefit to so many people I'd like to share them with you now:

Living the 6 Pillars to Optimum Health (6 Week Guided Program)

This amazing 6-week online and personally supported program will guide you through the process of *applying* the 6 Pillars of Optimum Health to your life. It will help you THRIVE, while establishing life-changing habits which will positively serve you for the rest of your life. The program will add energy and vitality to your life *right now*, and add months and years to your life. So if you'd like to go farther, deeper, faster (okay, not faster, how about more intensely) towards optimum health with me as your personal guide, for all the details check out:

www.theguidebooktooptimumhealth.com

The 30-Day Happiness Challenge

This unique 6-week coaching program is life changing. It consists of online and offline coaching tailored to your individual needs, PLUS 6 powerful one-on-one weekly coaching sessions which will teach you not only the foundational elements of health and happiness, but also techniques to develop the greatest habits of happiness, health, vitality, creativity, productivity and success. If you want to upgrade the course of your life, overcome challenges, achieve your biggest goals, and love the way you feel on a daily basis, this program is the game changer for you. For all the details check out:

www.30dayhappinesschallenge.com

7-Day Mind-Body Detox Retreats with Carl Massy

Ready? Set? DETOX! Join me for an amazing week getting squeaky clean inside. This is the kind of holistic mind, body, spirit detox retreat I always wanted for myself and had to create! I teach you the best daily practices I know. We eat the best food to cleanse your body. I run a series of powerful daily workshops to address all I know about happiness and health. There is yoga, meditation, energy altering guided meditations, reiki, physical detoxing, life master planning, relationship counselling 101, and the full-on opportunity to pick my brain (and mind) for one week. I would love to see you at one of the many detox retreats I run at various places throughout the world every year. For getting the jump on optimum health, addressing mid-life crisis or confusion, this retreat is ideal and the best investment you could make for your (glowing) future. For the details of the next location and dates, check out:

www.carlmassy.com/ training-events

Calling all health professionals... Workshops for Health, Fitness and Wellness

Take your practice—and yourself—to a whole new level of optimum functioning. Enhance your health, replenish your energy stores, rejuvenate your life, increase your knowledge, and enliven your commitment to helping others with my practical and transformative workshops for wellness professionals. Understand the body/mind/emotion connection more deeply to better serve your clients and meet their needs on a whole new plane. Increase their health potentials by learning practical tips, tools and strategies to make their life dreams (and yours) a reality. Specific case studies are examined to help understand the dynamics of why some people get great results and others don't, why some do the work and others can't, and what you can do to change the odds of their success more in their favor. Remember: Helping and loving yourself helps your clients change and love themselves.

BTW - I also run company and corporate workshops and seminars on health happiness, creativity and productivity. So if you think your workplace could benefit from a bit more fun and fulfillment (and whose couldn't?), drop my name to your HR department or send me an email direct and we'll come up with a master plan to get your company on board. I'm looking forward to seeing you soon!

Acknowledgements

As Hugh Grant found out in the movie *About a Boy*, it takes more than one person to create a meaningful life.

Life is about relationships and the relationships we have with people. And books are like life, created through relationships with any number of people, both directly and indirectly. At this point I'd like to briefly acknowledge the 'cool cats' in my life that helped make this book possible.

First and foremost there is Ferry Tan, my amazing partner, love of my life, and the person behind the boot that I occasionally and gratefully need up the backside every now and again when I forget to walk my own talk. Ferry believes in me more than I believe in myself sometimes, and is a big part of the reason I am where I am today. I'm so fortunate to have a partner who supports me so completely and tirelessly. She is also the creative genius behind the book's cover, all the illustrations and the entire layout (plus all my websites and online programs). She rocks!

The next person I want to high-five is Cate Montana, my amazing editor. She went WAY beyond the call of duty as an editor and added incredible and relevant content to help serve you in the best way possible. She did an impressive job, as an American, keeping my Aussie-isms under control, translating them into English where needed. So, thank you from the bottom of my heart.

I have had the support of some great teachers in the wellness field, whether through their written work or insightful teachings—special people like Dr.

Darren Weissman, Octavio Salvado, and Patty Tucker who have been extremely generous giving their time and energy sharing their wealth of knowledge so you could gain an even deeper understanding of how to get the most out of your life.

Thanks to a few of my great friends for supporting me emotionally and even financially to bring this book to fruition. Special thanks goes to Scot Braithwaite for his financial, business and emotional support, plus those long and investigative talks about the causes of illness in our modern lifestyles. Also a special mention to Troy Brice, an ex-Army classmate who has always had my back and who helped give me a leg up (and a room with an awesome view in Singapore) on many an occasion. To the Royal Military College Duntroon Class of 89, I thank you for your tolerance, the odd shove, encouragement, perspective and continued support over the last few decades. Thanks for helping me keep my feet on the ground, reminding me what is important in life.

A special thanks to great mentors, people and teachers Diane and Robert McCann who found time amongst their many life-changing retreats, courses and programs to share their years of experience in the wellness industry, helping me get back on the rails when I've had a train crash along the way. They help remind me that life (and success in this industry) is a journey that, like Rome, is not built in a day.

And finally, thanks to my awesome family. Thanks for helping shape me. Thanks for supporting me (long after I left home at 17). Thanks for teaching me values and virtues that serve me to this day.

Copyright

47736963R00162

Made in the USA
Charleston, SC
17 October 2015